plan to get
pregnant

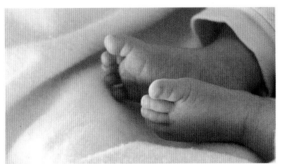

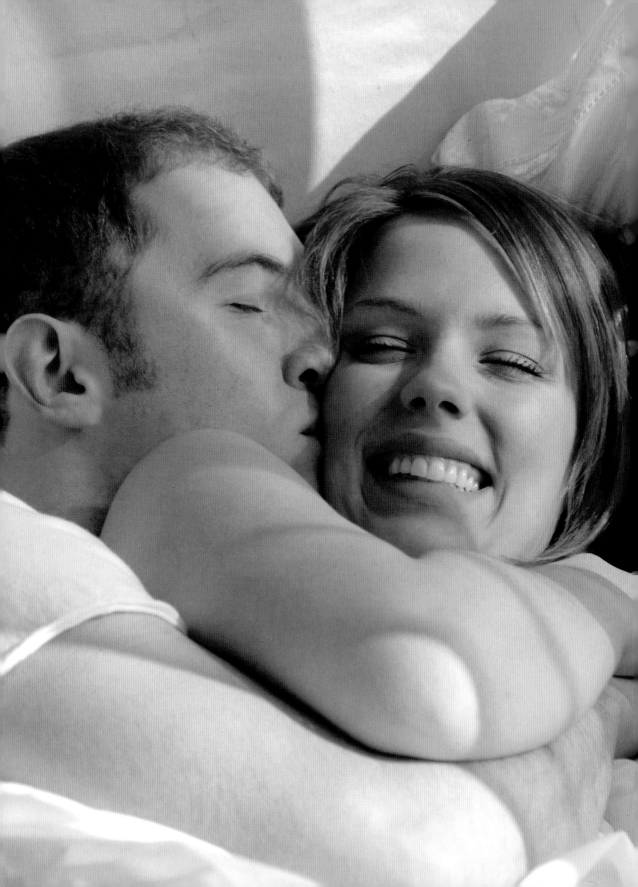

plan to get pregnant

pregnant

10 steps to **maximum fertility**

Zita West

LONDON, NEW YORK, MELBOURNE, MUNICH, and DELHI

Senior editor Esther Ripley
Project art editor Sara Kimmins
Editor Angela Baynham
Designer Ruth Hope
Production editor Jenny Woodcock
Production controller Hema Gohil
Managing editor Penny Warren
Managing art editor Marianne Markham
Picture research Jenny Baskaya
Jacket designer Sara Kimmins
Jacket editor Adam Powley
Illustrator Debbie Maizels
Creative technical support Sonia Charbonnier
Category publisher Peggy Vance, Corinne Roberts

First published in Great Britain in 2008
by Dorling Kindersley Limited,
80 Strand, London WC2R ORL
Penguin Group (UK)

4 6 8 10 9 7 5 3
016–AD366–March/08

A CIP catalogue record for this book is available from the British Library

ISBN: 978–1–4053–2052–8

Colour reproduced by MDP, UK
Printed and bound in China

Discover more at
www.dk.com

Contents

step**one**

This first step provides a general fertility check for couples planning to get pregnant, including how weight, age, medical history, and previous pregnancy complications might affect conception.

step**two**

Directed specifically at women, step two reveals all you need to know about female fertility, from analysis of your menstrual cycle and problems with periods to working out when you are at your most fertile and what happens at conception.

step**three**

Step three guides your male partner through all he needs to know about sperm production and semen analysis, and highlights the factors that might impact on his potential to father a child.

step**four**

Understanding sexual response and the factors that affect desire and libido is key to keeping your sex life spontaneous and passionate. This step addresses the problems that can arise with sex.

foreword

Depending on the source of evidence, between 10 and 20 per cent of couples will encounter difficulty in conceiving. Many of us believe that this percentage is unlikely to decline in the foreseeable future. Therefore many couples, and their parents, siblings and close friends, will need to seek advice about "what to do" to become parents.

The science of infertility has taken huge steps forward since the birth of Louise Brown, the world's first IVF baby, in 1978. In those days, IVF was regarded with suspicion by the medical profession and the media – some said it would never "catch on" and others that it was immoral, unethical and "against nature". Thirty years on, there are 3 million IVF children in the world and when yet another celebrity gives birth following IVF treatment it is no longer a headline-grabbing event in the tabloid press.

However, although the public seem to have accepted the realities of infertility treatment, we seem to have forgotten that having children is about much more than the act of sexual intercourse (or its laboratory equivalent). The value of this excellently produced guide to fertility, infertility, pregnancy and its problems lies in its holistic approach. Zita West has collected and interpreted information from the laboratory, from the clinic, and from practitioners of a great variety of complementary therapies and added a leavening of common sense to create a thoroughly readable guide to the maze of human reproductive biology and its malfunctions. She takes great care to remind couples who are struggling with infertility that they should continue to love and cherish each other and keep talking about and sympathizing with the stresses that investigations and treatment place on their relationship, to help them cope with the dehumanizing effects of intrusive and invasive treatments.

I was particularly pleased to see her emphasis on approaches to infertility other than IVF – many patients assume that they will need the "hi-tech" treatments so beloved of the media, when in fact they might be helped by simple advice on when to make love or by alteration in lifestyle. This is the beauty of Zita West's book, and where it stands out from its many competitors. Although she rightly spends time in considering the intricacies of IVF, she puts ART (Assisted Reproductive Technology) into context, highlighting means of self-help for couples and detailing the more gentle and possibly more acceptable approaches to conception. While the science of IVF is wondrous, going through the process in fertility clinics is less so. Reading this book will help many couples to cope better and come out of fertility treatment as healthy as when they entered it.

William L Ledger, Professor of Obstetrics and Gynaecology, University of Sheffield; Head of the Centre for Reproductive Medicine and Fertility, Jessop Wing, Royal Hallamshire Hospital, Sheffield.

introduction

"Whatever circumstances bring you to this book, my message is that you really can plan to get pregnant, taking it one step at a time. So much of your reproductive health is within your control, from improving your diet to revitalizing your sex life and dealing with life's emotional stresses"

The work I do every day at my clinic is aimed at helping couples understand how fertility works, not just from a physical perspective, but also emotionally and practically to give them the best chance of conceiving a baby. My clients range from those who have just come off the pill and need reassurance that everything is as it should be, through to couples with fertility issues who are preparing for some form of assisted conception.

No matter what stage they are at, I begin by looking at the complete picture of their life together to identify where changes might help improve their chances of conception. What I try to show is that many of the solutions they need are fairly simple to achieve. The great thing about the body is that it is always trying to regain its natural balance and by taking simples measures you can go a long way towards helping your body restore its equilibrium.

I find increasingly that for most busy working couples, life is permeated with stress. Their bodies are on high alert most of the time, and this is coupled with poor eating habits, long working hours, and lack of sleep. By the time they reach me, many couples are running on empty and it is no wonder that they are finding it harder to get pregnant. Their bodies are firing on all cylinders yet their reproductive health is something they have never taken a moment to consider.

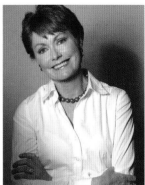

Everybody feels better when they have a plan to follow and at my clinic I use a programme of strategies and improvements supported by health-check and lifestyle questionnaires to help me identify where problems might lie. This book works in much the same way, with step-by-step plans for areas such as lifestyle, diet, and complementary therapies, backed with questionnaires that enable you to assess yourself and gain a greater understanding about what you need to do. Psychological and emotional factors in a relationship are often neglected topics in treatment-based fertility books, yet they can be a major factor in why couples are having difficulty becoming pregnant. In the step on sex and relationships, I emphasise that communication is the key – when a couple stops talking this is often when things start to go wrong.

Of course, getting pregnant is not the end of the journey, it's just the beginning. Staying pregnant and doing all you can to nurture yourself and your developing baby through pregnancy requires thought and planning too. My final step shows you how to make the best possible start.

Zita West

"As a **first step** I look at general **indicators of basic fertility** and assess any factors that might impact on the **ability to conceive**"

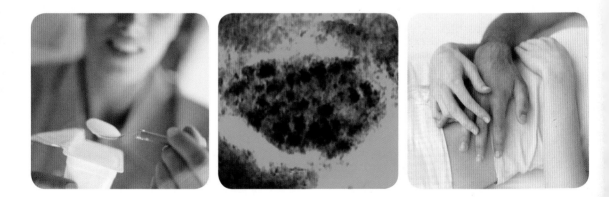

step**one**
trying for a baby

step one: **trying for a baby**

" In my **first consultation** with couples who are planning to get pregnant, I begin with a **fertility check** on factors such as age, health, and family history. This first step of the book takes a similar approach, helping you to assess where you stand **in terms of general fertility** before you attempt to **maximize your chances** of conceiving "

Q How does age affect fertility?

In women, age is the most important factor in determining fertility. A baby girl is born with around 1 million eggs; by puberty this ovarian reserve is down to less than half that number, and in the course of her reproductive life a woman will release only around 400 mature eggs. About 15 years before the menopause (from about the age of 35) her ovarian reserve declines further and the quality of her eggs is reduced. In some months an egg may not be produced at all. Despite all the medical advances in recent years, a woman cannot delay the age at which she reaches the menopause and therefore the age at which her fertility starts to diminish.

On pages 16 and 17, I provide more information on the so-called biological clock and on a woman's chance of conceiving at every stage of her reproductive life. I also explain the significance of the male partner's age in how fertile a couple is likely to be. This is important because we now know that in around 40 per cent of cases infertility is due to the male partner, and in a high proportion of those, age is the main factor.

It is easy to dwell on the negative aspects of age and to become demoralized by the statistics, but if age is likely to be an issue for you, stay positive – I regularly see and successfully treat many women over the age of 35. Bear

in mind that, on average, it takes between 6 and 12 months to conceive across all couples, regardless of age. I also believe that there is a lot you can do to make sure you give yourself the best chance of becoming pregnant. For example, lifestyle and nutrition have an influence on fertility, and these are discussed in detail in Steps 5 and 6.

However, if you are over 35, and you have been having targeted intercourse for more than six months, you should consider having some fertility tests to rule out any underlying problems.

Q Can I check my ovarian reserve?

In the past, one of the difficulties for a woman was trying to assess how many fertile years she had ahead of her, given that she ceases to be fertile several years before her periods actually stop. Now, a testing kit called Plan Ahead, which can be bought over the counter, has become available. This measures three hormones in the blood – inhibin B, AMH (anti-mullerian hormone), and follicle-stimulating hormone (FSH) – using a blood sample taken by a GP or nurse on the second or third day of the menstrual cycle. The kit is then posted to the manufacturer's laboratory where the blood is analysed, and the level of hormones detected determines the ovarian reserve.

Although the test can undoubtedly be useful, for example in assessing whether it might be worth embarking on IVF sooner rather than later, it is important to understand that your ovarian reserve is only one of many factors that influence your fertility and chances of conception. The test will not tell you, for example, if you have blocked fallopian tubes or whether your partner has a low sperm count. Whatever the results, I would advise you to seek professional help to discuss your own personal situation.

> ## Zita's **tip**
> If you think either you or your partner have a **fertility problem**, consult your doctor now.

Q I am overweight. Will this impact on my chances of conceiving?

Women who are significantly overweight can find it harder to become pregnant. This is because fat cells release oestrogen, which in turn tells the pituitary gland to suppress the release of follicle-stimulating hormone (FSH). Without FSH, ovulation does not occur (see pages 36–37 for more on the hormonal cycle). If your body mass index (BMI – see below) is over 30, you are considered to be clinically obese and this can lead to a whole range of medical problems that can reduce fertility. One of the most common of these is polycystic ovary syndrome (PCOS – see page 22), but you will also be at risk of developing diabetes, heart disease, and high blood pressure, all of which can harm you and your baby.

Being overweight also has an impact on male fertility. Men tend to carry extra weight around their abdomen and genital area. This can cause an increase in temperature and therefore affect sperm production.

If you are overweight, speak to your GP or a nutritionist about the best way to lose weight safely (see also Step 6). You might only need to lose a small amount to restore your hormonal balance and improve your fertility.

Q Does it matter if I am underweight?

Women who have too little body fat can find that their oestrogen levels fall and this can lead to their periods becoming irregular or stopping altogether. So, if your BMI is under 20, you need to find a way to put on some weight in order to restore your hormonal balance. Talk to a nutritionist and/or a counsellor if you need help with this.

Furthermore, it is important to develop good dietary habits before you become pregnant because once you do conceive, the first three months of the pregnancy are critical in the development of your baby. That is when all the building blocks are put in place for your baby's organs, including bones, heart, and brain, so your body needs to be able to nourish the developing fetus.

find out more: **bmi and body shape**

A woman's weight can be a significant cause of fertility problems. The best way to determine whether you are underweight or overweight is to calculate your body mass index (BMI), which is used by health professionals to determine whether or not an individual's weight falls within acceptable limits. This is done using a

simple formula (see below). The ideal BMI is between 20 and 25; outside this range your weight could be having a negative effect on your fertility. There is no hard and fast rule about what level your BMI needs to reach for it to start to impact on your chances of getting pregnant, but these figures should act as a guide to help you see if you could have a weight problem.

To find your BMI, divide your weight in kilos by the square of your height in metres. Here is a calculation for a woman who is 1.7m (5ft 7in) tall, weighing 65kg (9st 11lb):

1.7 x 1.7 = 2.89

65kg divided by 2.89 = 22.5

Her BMI is 22.5 and therefore falls within the acceptable range.

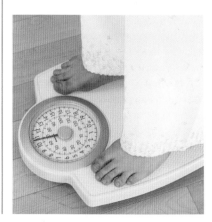

Weight is used in the calculation of body mass index and helps to establish whether or not fertility might be at risk.

are you an **apple** or a **pear shape**?

It seems that women who carry excess abdominal weight (apple shaped) can be less fertile than women whose excess weight is distributed around their hips and bottom (pear shaped). The reasons for this are not totally understood, but one Dutch study has shown that there is a clear link between women's body shapes and conception rates.

Q When was your last smear test?

It is really important that you have a smear test regularly and certainly before you start trying to get pregnant. If a test shows that there are precancerous cell changes, and you are already pregnant, you need to be monitored carefully and will have to wait until after you have had your baby before you can be treated. The NHS screens women every three years, but increasingly women are choosing to have annual smear tests done privately.

Q Do you know whether or not you are rubella immune?

Ninety per cent of women are immune to rubella (also known as German measles) because they were immunized against it during childhood. If you were not, you should consider getting immunized now, and then avoid conceiving for three months. If you do catch the virus in the early stages of a pregnancy, this has potentially serious consequences for the baby you are carrying: if you contract rubella in the first eight weeks of pregnancy, you run an increased risk of miscarriage; if you contract it in the first 12 weeks, your baby has an 80 per cent risk of congenital abnormalities that include deafness, eye cataracts, and heart defects; if it is between 13 and 17 weeks, your baby still runs the risk of being born deaf.

Sadly, the recent loss of public confidence concerning the MMR vaccine has meant that in some parts of the UK the percentage of children immunized against rubella has fallen significantly, and this has increased the risk of a non-rubella-immune woman catching the virus from infected children when she is pregnant. So do get your rubella status checked before trying to conceive. The only way to do this is with a blood test.

Q Did your mother suffer from an early menopause?

Early menopause occurs when a woman's periods stop before the age of 40. This condition, also known as premature ovarian failure (POF – see page 22), can be hereditary, so if your mother suffered from this, you should bear it in mind when you are thinking of getting pregnant. Also remember that, as with the normal menopause, a woman with POF will stop producing fertilizable eggs several years (potentially up to 10) before her periods stop.

> **Zita's tip**
> **Be prepared** for pregnancy: check your **rubella status** and make sure your **smear test** is up to date.

Q Have you or your partner ever been treated for cancer?

Fortunately, many people now make a full recovery from cancer, but if either you or your partner have had treatment that involved radiation to the abdomen or pelvic area and/or chemotherapy, it is possible that, despite the best endeavours of the medical staff, fertility has been affected. For men as much as for women, it very much depends on the dose and type of drug given. Speak to a specialist to find out more.

Women whose cancer was treated before the age of 30 have the best chance of subsequently getting pregnant, although I have seen many women over this age conceive. For men, a sperm test would be necessary to determine whether or not sperm production had resumed after treatment – it can take up to four years for this to happen.

When cancer is diagnosed it is worth talking to your specialist about the possibility of harvesting and freezing eggs and sperm, before treatment begins. Freezing of embryos has been available for some time, but an increasing number of units now have the technology to perform these procedures with individual eggs and sperm.

Q I have had abdominal surgery. Will this affect my fertility?

If you are in doubt about any abdominal surgery that you or your partner have undergone, you should consult your doctor and ask to be referred for specific tests. See page 52 in Step 3 for more information on whether sperm production can be affected by previous abdominal surgery.

Conditions such as burst appendix, endometriosis (where tissue that normally lines the uterus attaches to other organs in the abdomen – see page 22), or Crohn's disease (an inflammatory disease of the digestive tract) may require surgery, which can affect a woman's fertility because of the risk of adhesions (scar tissue) forming in the abdominal cavity.

Q What **contraception** have you been using?

It is possible that contraceptive methods you have used in the past may have affected your fertility. Ask your GP about tests if you suspect there might be a problem.

The pill I find that it is not unusual for women to go on the pill at 16, then come off it 15 years later with the intention of starting a family, only to discover that they have little idea how long their body will take to get back to normal hormonally. Women used to be advised to wait three months after coming off the pill before trying to conceive, but research now indicates that this is not necessary and that, in fact, the body is more fertile immediately after stopping the pill, because that is the time when there is a big hormonal push. After this surge, it can then take a while – possibly up to 18 months – for the hormonal balance to be restored, so conception can be delayed. This is especially the case if you have been taking the combined (oestrogen/progestogen) pill as opposed to the progestogen-only pill (progestogen is the synthetic form of the hormone progesterone).

The progestogen component of the pill causes changes in your cervical secretions and when you stop taking it these secretions may need to return to normal so that they can create a sperm-friendly environment. That said, there is no reason to delay trying to get pregnant when coming off the pill.

Contraception injections This form of hormonal contraception – of which Depo Provera is the best known – is given via a three-monthly injection. If you are trying for a baby it is quite common to take 12 months or more to conceive after the last injection, since the effects of the injection, which include changes in your mucus pattern, can continue beyond the three-month interval. If necessary, use a different method of contraception, such as a condom, to delay conception to an appropriate time after your last injection.

Intrauterine device (IUD) or coil There is an increased risk of pelvic inflammatory disease (PID – see page 18) for women fitted with an IUD and this can subsequently affect their fertility. However, the risks are

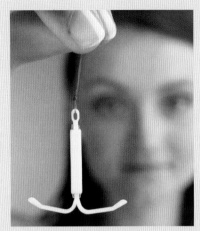

The Mirena coil is a progestogen-releasing contraceptive device. When you are ready for pregnancy, ask your doctor to remove it. Your menstrual cycle will return to normal over the next few months.

strongly related to lifestyle, so women who are fitted with an IUD and are in a long-term relationship with one partner are at very low risk. Also, the new IUDs further reduce the likelihood of PID occurring, as does the Mirena progestogen-releasing intrauterine system, because it thickens the cervical mucus.

Implants These prevent ovulation by the slow release of progestogen from a match-sized rod implanted under the skin. As with other forms of hormonal contraception, the cervical mucus is also affected, and it can take a little while for this to return to normal and for hormonal balance to be fully restored.

There are other ways of delivering hormonal contraception, such as using an intrauterine system (see above) or a contraceptive patch (containing oestrogen and progestogen). If you use one of these methods, you should discuss the expected time for return of fertility with your contraceptive provider.

Condom This has no effect on future fertility. However, your sexual health was protected when you were using a condom, so once you stop using this form of contraception, you need to ensure that you do not put yourself at risk of catching a sexually transmitted infection (chlamydia, for example) that could harm your fertility (see pages 18–19).

find out more: **the ticking clock**

In the UK, the **average age** to have a first child is now **just over 29**, up from 26 in the early 1980s, despite the fact that our bodies have not changed.

Biologically, the best years for a woman to have a baby are between the ages of 20 and 25. That is when women are at their most fertile and their bodies are fully grown and in their prime. Before that, problems caused by pregnancy are often more emotional than physical. After the age of 30, fertility begins to decline, slowly at first, then sharply from the age of 35, while beyond 40 the ability to conceive is severely reduced.

I would urge you to consider two things when you are planning a family. First, there is never a right time to have a baby. Yes, your life will change, but you should not assume that you will not be able to cope if the baby arrives at a time when you do not feel ready. Secondly, think about how many children you might like to have. If the answer is more than one, you need to consider how big a gap you would like to have between them. If you are over 35, you might not want to wait too long between pregnancies.

conception **timescale**

- One study showed that 75 per cent of women aged 30 who are trying to conceive go on to start a successful pregnancy within one year.
- By the time they are 35, that figure has fallen to 66 per cent.
- For those aged 40, it is down to 44 per cent.
- By age 45, pregnancy has become very difficult to achieve.

age and risk of abnormality

The older a woman is, the older her eggs are and the more likely it is that when fertilized they will contain an abnormal number of chromosomes. Once she reaches her mid-30s there is an increasingly high risk of her having a child with a congenital abnormality, which means that the baby is born with a disorder or problem. Most often, this is because there are too few or too many of a particular chromosome. Trisomies occur when there are three copies of a chromosome, instead of the normal pair. The most common of these is Down's syndrome, or trisomy 21, in which there are three copies of chromosome 21.

It also appears that the man's age affects the risk if both partners are over 35 years and increases the incidence of babies born with certain congenital defects. A severe defect is the most common cause of miscarriage, the rate of which is much higher in women over 35 (see page 26).

risk of chromosomal abnormalities						
maternal age at delivery date	30	35	38	42	44	46
risk of Down's syndrome	1 in 952	1 in 385	1 in 175	1 in 64	1 in 38	1 in 23
risk of any abnormality at birth	1 in 384	1 in 204	1 in 103	1 in 40	1 in 25	1 in 15

the male factor

Men's fertility is also known to decline with age, although not to the same extent as women's. According to one study, women who are aged 35 to 39 are 10 per cent less likely in any given cycle to achieve conception with a man who is five years older than them, than with one who is the same age. This is because as men get older, their sperm's volume, structure (whether or not they are healthy and undamaged), and motility (their ability to arrive at their destination) goes down (see Step 3).

The age of the male partner can also be a problem for reasons that are not necessarily physical. If your partner is significantly older than you, for example, it may be that he already has a family, and issues can arise from this. Conversely, he might be younger and not ready, perhaps psychologically, to have children. In both cases, this can end up putting a strain on your relationship and making it more difficult for you to conceive. In any event, if your age difference is causing problems, it is vital you address the issue, either by talking things through with your partner or by seeking professional help together.

abnormal sperm in **men over 45:**

16%

compared to 4 per cent for those in their late 20s. Men aged 45 years or older face a five-fold increase in the time taken to achieve a pregnancy compared with men less than 30 years old (32 months versus six months).

can science defy age?

The commonly held view that "you can always get pregnant with IVF" if you fail to conceive naturally is a misconception, even though I am the first to applaud the fact that, thankfully, there are many ways in which modern medicine can now help infertile couples to become parents. Only half the women who postpone pregnancy for the first time from 30 to 35, and less than 30 per cent of those who postpone it from 35 to 40 will be helped.

case**study**

Susan and Jeff were both 39 when they came to me looking for advice. They had been trying to conceive for nine months.

Susan Because I came from a big family (I have six brothers and sisters) I always thought I would get pregnant very easily, so I started to get a bit nervous when nothing had happened after nine months of trying. Both Jeff and I made big changes to our diet. We stopped eating any processed foods and made an effort to eat as much fruit and vegetables as possible. We both stopped drinking alcohol. Although I am 39, I'm fit and healthy and I exercise three or four times a week.

We decided to arrange a consultation with Zita because I needed some reassurance that everything was fine with our fertility. She arranged for us both to have some tests done and it did come as quite a shock when the results showed that my levels of the hormone FSH were slightly raised and to learn that this was possibly a sign

that the menopause is approaching. On top of that, Jeff's sperm count was low.

I had always hoped to conceive naturally, but when Zita explained that despite being fit and healthy our ages were working against us, I realized we didn't have the time we had thought we might have to keep on trying. On taking advice we decided to opt for an assisted fertility route. I know there can be no guarantees, but I don't want to waste any further time and end up looking back with regrets.

It is difficult to say how long you can afford to keep trying to conceive naturally, but in this instance we all agreed the best way forward was to start IVF treatment straight away.

Q How do **sexually transmitted infections** affect a couple's plans for getting pregnant?

I often recommend that my patients – both male and female – go for a sexual health test either at their local hospital (at the genito-urinary medicine clinic) or at a private clinic because a previously untreated sexually transmitted infection (STI) can be a cause of infertility. It seems obvious, but it is still worth pointing out that a man who suffers from an infection could either be harming his own future fertility, if he develops prostatitis (inflammation of the prostate gland), for example, or his partner's fertility if he infects her. The same applies if a woman infects her partner.

Sexually transmitted infections are often symptomless. This is why it is important to be screened so that, if necessary, you can be diagnosed and treated as early as possible, and before the infection starts to affect your chances of conceiving. Also, treatment during pregnancy is more difficult, and the presence of an STI can affect your baby and cause premature birth. Antibiotics are the most common form of treatment for STIs.

Chlamydia and gonorrhoea You might think that you would know if you had ever contracted an STI such as chlamydia or gonorrhoea but this is not necessarily the case. Chlamydia, for example, is the most common sexually transmitted infection in the UK, and is usually symptomless, particularly in women. Yet it is thought that 15 to 20 per cent of the sexually active population could have been infected. Furthermore, it is estimated that 10 to 40 per cent of women with untreated chlamydia go on to develop pelvic inflammatory disease (PID) – see right.

In women, if it is not treated early, the infection can spread to the fallopian tubes and cause blockage, which in turn can lead to infertility or an ectopic pregnancy. In men, untreated chlamydia can cause damage to the sperm-carrying tubes and ducts in the testes and this can result in blockage and therefore infertility.

Gonorrhoea is highly contagious, and unprotected sex with an infected person transmits the infection in 90 per cent of cases. Twice as many men as women are infected. Like chlamydia, this bacterial infection is often

symptoms of an **STI** may include:

- Abnormal and often smelly discharge from the vagina or penis
- Abdominal pain
- A burning sensation when passing urine
- Flu-like feeling and a high fever

symptomless, but it can produce an unpleasant vaginal discharge and abdominal and urinary pain. Untreated gonorrhoea often leads to pelvic inflammatory disease and blocked fallopian tubes (see below). Men show symptoms including discharge, abdominal pain, and a high fever.

Pelvic inflammatory disease (PID) This occurs when an untreated STI (often chlamydia) spreads up through the cervix and into the uterus, fallopian tubes, and pelvis. PID often causes painful intercourse but the disease can be symptomless and some women don't realize there is a problem until they try to conceive. The infection itself is easily treated with antibiotics. However, if left untreated for some time, it can cause scarring or even blockage to

Dye shows up narrowing and distortion of the fallopian tube

Uterus

Blocked fallopian tube cannot be seen because no dye can enter it

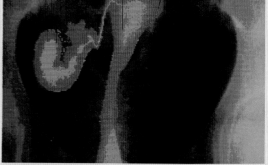

PID is diagnosed by introducing contrast dye into the uterus. Here, one fallopian tube is distorted, the other blocked.

the fallopian tubes. If that is the case, your fertility will be affected and you will run a greater risk of having an ectopic pregnancy (see page 26). Surgery would be necessary to remove the blockage.

Herpes This is a common STI but one that very few people openly admit to having contracted. The herpes simplex virus is dormant in the majority of the population, so they probably don't even know they carry it. There are two types of herpes viruses: type 1 (HSV1) causes cold sores; type 2 (HSV2) causes genital herpes. If you contract HSV2 the initial infection is usually the worst, producing flu-like symptoms, a burning sensation around the genitalia, aching legs, and genital sores or blisters that are uncomfortable and itchy. You are contagious for around five days after the sores have crusted over, which in itself can take a week. Once you are infected, subsequent flare-ups tend to occur during times where your immunity is under attack: when you are unwell, tired, or under stress, for example. Women can also find that hormonal changes set off an attack around the time of menstruation. If you are getting regular attacks you will not be able to have unprotected sex, and so are limiting the times when you can conceive. In other respects, herpes does not compromise your fertility.

Trichomoniasis This STI, caused by the organism *Trichomonas vaginalis*, doesn't cause PID. However, as well as causing an itching and burning sensation in the vagina and urethra (and, for men, pain when urinating), it changes the consistency of the cervical mucus, making it difficult for sperm to get through. As a result, fertility may be affected.

Bacterial vaginosis: mycoplasmosis, ureaplasmosis, gardnerella These bacterial infections are caused by microscopic organisms – *Mycoplasma hominis*, *Ureaplasma urealyticum*, and *Gardnerella vaginalis* – found in the genito-urinary tracts of men and women. They are normally harmless, and although they are not STIs as such they sometimes proliferate and can be transmitted from one partner to another. These organisms, which are often symptomless, are found in higher concentrations in couples who are having trouble conceiving. They may also be linked to the presence of another STI. Although they do not lead to PID in women, they are thought to raise the

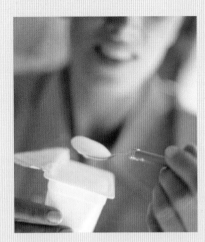

Eating "live" natural yogurt helps to treat candida by restoring the natural flora in the gut.

chance of miscarriage, and men with mycoplasmosis have increased numbers of abnormal sperm. Because they are not routinely tested for on the NHS, you might think about paying to get yourself screened for these infections if you have been trying unsuccessfully to conceive for a while or have recently suffered a miscarriage. A short course of antibiotics normally clears up these infections within a couple of days, although the conditions do tend to recur.

Candida Although not an STI, a common condition that primarily affects the vaginal secretions is *Candida*, also known as vaginal thrush. If you notice that your secretions have become smelly or are making you feel itchy or uncomfortable, consult your doctor, as you may have developed thrush and it could be making it harder for you to conceive. Thrush (sometimes referred to as a yeast infection) occurs when the naturally occurring yeast, *Candida albicans*, which is present in our bodies, proliferates. If left untreated, it can impact on your health in general, making you feel very tired and run down and damaging your absorption of essential nutrients. Candida thrives on a poor diet that is high in refined sugar, so one of the easiest ways to cure this condition (as well as using anti-fungal creams or pessaries) and to prevent its return is to eat healthily and cut out refined sugars wherever possible. Eating "live" natural yogurt containing *Lactobacillus acidophilus* also helps to restore the natural flora in the gut.

Q Which medical conditions can affect fertility?

There is now a greater awareness that many women who are having trouble getting or staying pregnant are in fact suffering from some sort of autoimmune disorder, such as rheumatoid arthritis or certain forms of thyroid disease or lupus. These are thought to contribute to a significant proportion of what is called "unexplained infertility", where no obvious cause is found, and of recurrent miscarriage, where the woman has three or more consecutive pregnancy losses. The following three questions and answers give more detailed information on each of these conditions.

Q I've been told I have an underactive thyroid. Will this cause problems with conception?

The thyroid gland, situated in the middle of the lower neck, below the Adam's apple, produces hormones that are essential in regulating the physiological and metabolic functions in your body, including those that are part of reproduction. Thyroid disease affects around 5 per cent of women, half of whom suffer from an underactive thyroid gland (hypothyroidism), while the other half suffer from an overactive thyroid (hyperthyroidism).

Hypothyroidism is much more of a problem for fertility and may cause anovulation (no eggs are released), luteal phase defect (see page 38), and hyperprolactinemia (excessive levels of the hormone prolactin). It can occur either because the thyroid gland doesn't produce enough

of the hormone thyroxine, or because the feedback mechanism that "instructs" the gland to produce more thyroxine fails to function properly, or because the body is not able to use the hormone correctly. Hypothyroidism can also be caused by an autoimmune condition where the body produces antibodies that attack its own tissue, in this case the thyroid gland itself. This then affects the thyroid's ability to produce hormones, which hinders fertility and leads to a higher risk of miscarriage once a woman is pregnant.

Thyroid disorders are often diagnosed with a simple blood test, and treatment usually involves straightforward medication. Your doctor will then advise you on regulating the dose while you are trying to become pregnant and once you have conceived. Complementary therapies cannot affect the actual hormone imbalance caused by the malfunctioning thyroid gland, so they should never replace conventional drugs. However, diet and lifestyle can help to manage the effects of an underactive thyroid (see Step 6).

If undiagnosed or left untreated, both hypothyroidism and hyperthyroidism increase the risk of miscarriage, as well as affecting fertility.

Q I have lupus. How will this affect my plans to get pregnant?

Lupus, or systemic lupus erythematosus (SLE), is an autoimmune disease that causes inflammation and damage to various body tissues, leading to painful or swollen joints and skin rashes, among other symptoms. Treatment is often in the form of corticosteroids, so pregnancy counselling and planning are very important. Ideally, you should be symptom-free and not taking medication for six months before you conceive.

Women suffering from lupus are at higher risk of miscarriage, particularly those who have tested positive for antiphospholipid antibodies (APAs) or anti-nuclear antibodies (ANAs). Fortunately, with correct diagnosis, and even though the pregnancy is considered high risk, most of these women now go on to carry their babies safely to term. Regular care and good nutrition during pregnancy are essential because lupus sufferers are more likely to develop high blood pressure, diabetes, and kidney complications.

Some women may experience a mild to moderate flare-up during or after pregnancy, but it is really important that you are under the care of a specialist during your pregnancy, so that complications can be spotted early and managed quickly.

symptoms of **thyroid** problems

It is important to be aware that symptoms for thyroid disease are very varied and can easily be mistaken for other disorders.

hypothyroidism	hyperthyroidism
▪ extreme tiredness	▪ weight loss
▪ poor tolerance of cold	▪ feeling very hot
▪ weight gain or loss	▪ excessive sweating
▪ poor appetite	▪ menstrual problems
▪ dry skin and hair	▪ joint pains
▪ menstrual problems	▪ hand tremors

Q Does rheumatoid arthritis have any impact on fertility or pregnancy?

Rheumatoid arthritis (RA), another one of the autoimmune conditions, does impact on fertility in that it may increase the risk of miscarriage through the production of autoantibodies such as antiphospholipid antibodies (APAs), which sometimes attack the body's own tissues. RA occurs in around 1 in every 1,500 pregnancies, and as with other autoimmune disorders, pregnancy improves the condition for many women, though they often relapse a few months after giving birth. A specialist will determine which drugs are safe to use for treatment of RA during pregnancy.

Q Does diabetes reduce fertility?

Type 1 diabetes develops if the body is unable to produce any insulin and usually appears before the age of 40. Type 2 diabetes occurs when the body can make insulin but not enough, or the insulin that is produced is not effective. This is often linked with being overweight and tends to develop in people over the age of 40._ Whether or not you have type 1 or type 2 diabetes, and whether or not you are insulin-dependent, if you control your condition well, your fertility will not be affected. However, if your diabetes is poorly controlled and you regularly have high blood glucose levels, your ovulation may be affected and it will be harder to get pregnant.

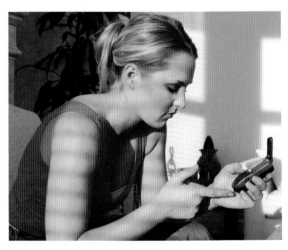

In most cases diabetes is well controlled and should not have any detrimental effect on a woman's ability to conceive.

Women who are diabetic do have an increased risk of pregnancy complications, miscarriage, or of having a baby with severe congenital anomalies including heart and neural tube defects. It is therefore vital that you control your blood sugar levels and this can be done by eating the right foods and taking certain nutritional supplements such as folic acid (see Step 6). Speak to your specialist to make sure you are doing all you can to control your condition.

For men, this condition is not thought to harm their sperm production, but up to 25 per cent of long-standing diabetics (of 10 years or more) are known to experience erectile dysfunction (see page 72).

Q I think I might be anaemic. Will this affect my chances of conceiving?

Every cell in your body needs an adequate supply of oxygen, which is carried by the pigment haemoglobin in red blood cells. Anaemia occurs when there is a lack of red blood cells in your body. The most common cause of anaemia is a lack of iron, which is needed for the production of haemoglobin. Other types of anaemia include folic acid deficiency anaemia and pernicious anaemia (vitamin B12 deficiency).

It is much harder to conceive if you are anaemic as your body is already having to work harder to get sufficient oxygen to its vital organs, let alone the reproductive organs. In addition, if you are anaemic you are likely to suffer from irregular menstrual cycles, and anaemia can also interfere with ovulation.

Symptoms of anaemia include heavy periods, constant tiredness, breathlessness, pale skin, dizziness, and recurrent infections. If you suffer from these you should go to your doctor who will do a simple blood test to analyse your haemoglobin levels. In a healthy female these should be 11 to 15.

Iron supplements are usually prescribed, but it can take up to six weeks for the blood to recover. Eating foods rich in iron, such as eggs, fish, poultry, green leafy vegetables, and liver can help. Foods rich in vitamin B12 include lamb, sardines, and salmon. Foods rich in folic acid include dark green leafy vegetables, salmon, avocados, whole grains, and pulses. Vitamin C can improve iron absorption, whereas dairy-rich products can limit it.

Women with malabsorption problems, such as coeliac disease, or who suffer from heavy periods are particularly prone to anaemia, as are frequent dieters and vegetarians.

Q What are the most common **medical causes** of female infertility?

When physical problems occur within the female reproductive system, they can make it more difficult to conceive.

Polycystic ovary syndrome (PCOS) This condition occurs when the ovaries develop lots of tiny cysts on the surface. These contain egg follicles that have not matured properly due to a complex hormonal imbalance, with the result that ovulation is affected and fertility significantly impaired. PCOS affects 5 to 10 per cent of women in the Western world.

Symptoms include greasy skin, irregular or absent periods, increased facial hair, weight gain (and difficulty losing it), difficulty getting pregnant, and recurrent miscarriage. If your mother or sister had/has PCOS, you may have a genetic predisposition to the condition. Women who are overweight are also more at risk.

If you suffer from PCOS, you may be given a hormone treatment to rebalance your hormones and improve ovulation. However, if you are overweight, you may find that you can improve your condition significantly simply by losing weight. Even a 10 per cent reduction in weight could balance your hormones

sufficiently to restore your fertility. Aim for a slow weight-loss programme involving a low GI (glycaemic index) diet that includes lots of complex carbohydrates (see Step 6). These keep your blood sugar levels even, your glucose levels down, and your insulin production at the correct level. Stress-relieving complementary therapies, such as yoga, relaxation techniques, and acupuncture, may also help boost fertility (see Step 8).

Endometriosis This is a highly complex medical condition that occurs when endometrial tissue from the lining of the uterus "migrates" to other parts of the pelvic region, such as the ovaries, fallopian tubes, or bladder. The tissue responds to hormonal changes and therefore bleeds at the same time as your period. This eventually leads to scarring and adhesions. Endometriosis is a major cause of failure to conceive.

Symptoms include severe menstrual cramps, long heavy periods (including clots), and pain during intercourse. Having an immediate family member affected by the condition also raises your likelihood of developing it.

It is possible to become pregnant if you suffer from mild endometriosis, but if it is moderate or severe, you may need

Ovary *Cystic follicles on ovary surface*

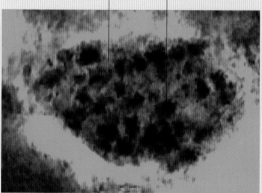

This ultrasound scan reveals PCOS. Multiple cysts (black) have formed on the ovary surface.

Endometriotic spots

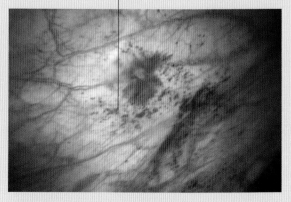

These spots seen in the abdominal cavity are a clear indication of endometriosis, which is a major cause of failure to conceive.

some form of medical treatment (which could include surgery) to improve your chance of conceiving. However, changes to your diet may also improve some of your symptoms and reduce the severity of the condition (see Step 6). Certain complementary therapies, including acupuncture, may also help (see pages 134–135).

Fibroids These benign tumours grow in the uterine cavity inside or outside the uterus. They are very common (as many as 20 to 50 per cent of women aged between 35 and 50 are thought to have them) and in many cases they don't harm a woman's chances of getting pregnant. Often, the presence of fibroids produces no symptoms at all, although some women do experience pain, heavy or irregular bleeding, and menstrual cramps.

Fibroids may impact on fertility if they are on the outside of the uterus preventing the fallopian tube from retrieving an egg after ovulation. If they are growing on the wall of the uterus, they may interfere with the embryo's ability to implant in the uterine lining. Larger fibroids (4–5cm/1½–2in in diameter) can cause problems in later pregnancy.

Fibroids may be treated with conventional medicine (including surgery) but as they are oestrogen-sensitive, a low-fat, high-fibre diet can also help. (Fat cells stimulate oestrogen production, so reducing fat intake will reduce your levels of that hormone). Acupuncture and reflexology may also help (see Steps 6 and 8).

Fibroid

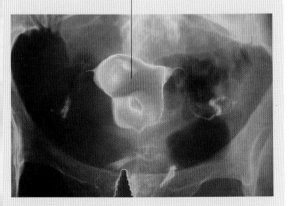

This X-ray of a woman's uterus, highlighted using radio opaque material, shows a fibroid growing on the internal wall.

Q Can a previous termination (abortion) have an effect?

The decision to terminate a pregnancy, for whatever reason, is rarely taken lightly. Nowadays, such a procedure is invariably safe: only 0.5 per cent of women find that they are unable to conceive following a termination and this is usually because they contracted an infection at or soon after the procedure. In the many cases, having a termination has no physical impact on a woman's future fertility and does not increase her chance of miscarriage.

However, in my experience, for some women a termination can leave a psychological mark for many years to come – sometimes without the woman being aware of it – and as such can interfere with her subsequent ability to get pregnant. I regularly see women who believe that they have dealt with the psychological repercussions of a termination they had when they were younger. Yet, when we discuss things in more depth, they realize that, in fact, they have not come to terms with their decision and this could be stopping them from accepting another pregnancy. This can be particularly difficult to deal with if the pregnancy that was terminated was with the current partner. Once these women have acknowledged their feelings, they are often able to "let go" and move on to conceiving another child.

Q I've had a D&C. Does this reduce my chances of conceiving?

D&C (dilation and curettage) is a procedure in which the neck of the uterus is dilated (widened) and a sample of the uterine lining is scraped away for analysis. Rest assured that, unless you were very unlucky and contracted a post-surgery infection or Asherman's syndrome (scar tissue in the uterus), which may have caused tubal damage, the procedure itself will have had no impact on your chances of conceiving.

Zita's **tip**

Many of the **medical causes** of infertility can be diagnosed fairly easily and **treated effectively**.

Q Are you taking **regular medication**?

I am listing below some of the more common forms of medication and describing how they might affect your chances of getting pregnant. For men, certain medications and medical conditions affect sperm count or can cause erectile problems and these are dealt with in Step 3. This list cannot cover the impact on fertility for every drug for every medical condition that you might suffer from, nor whether that drug is or isn't safe to use during pregnancy.

Clearly, if you suffer from a specific or chronic medical condition, it is essential that you take the drugs you have been prescribed, but it is important to be aware of the possible side effects for your fertility. If either you or your partner has a known medical condition (that may or may not require prescribed medication), you should be discussing the potential impact of your condition and the medication you take with your GP or specialist.

In addition, any illness or prescribed medication can have an effect on cervical secretions (see page 40) – be aware of this so that you can anticipate changes and observe any variations.

The information I give here has been divided into two tables: the first covers some of the most common, over-the-counter drugs and their effects on fertility; the second covers medication that is given only on prescription. In both tables, I have also indicated where a drug is known to have a harmful effect on certain aspects of nutrition, so that you are aware of the impact a drug–nutrient interaction can have on your diet (see Step 6).

over-the-counter medication

drug	taken for	effect on fertility or nutrition
Ibuprofen	General pain relief, including period pains, back pain, headaches	Ibuprofen is a non-steroidal anti-inflammatory drug (NSAID) and can affect ovulation and implantation and may increase the risk of miscarriage.
Aspirin	General pain relief, including period pains, back pain, headaches	Also a NSAID, aspirin (which thins the blood) might reduce fertility by affecting implantation, although baby aspirin may be used under GP supervision to enhance implantation for women with certain blood disorders.
Paracetamol	General pain relief, including period pains, back pain, headaches	Paracetamol does not have anti-inflammatory properties and has no known effect on fertility.
Antihistamines such as *Piriton* and *Sudafed*	Allergies, coughs, colds	These can dry or thicken cervical secretions and reduce quantity and may also interfere with implantation.
Antacid medication such as *Gaviscon*	Digestive disorders	Depending on the amount taken, these can affect absorption of iron, which can lead to anaemia and can harm fertility (see page 21).
Laxatives	Constipation	Nutritional effect: can hinder absorption of calcium, which is essential for the production of healthy eggs and sperm.

prescribed medication

drug	taken for	effect on fertility or nutrition
Isotretinoin	Acne	It is vital to get advice from your doctor if you are taking this drug. It can reduce and dry up cervical secretions and carries a high risk of birth defects.
Inhaled bronchodilators such as *Ventolin* (salbutamol)	Asthma	These are used to relieve symptoms and are generally safe, but discuss with your doctor nonetheless.
Steroids taken in tablet form, such as cortisone and prednisolone	Rheumatoid arthritis, lupus, severe respiratory or skin conditions	Taken long term, steroids can cause a problem as they can delay ovulation and may cause irregular menstrual bleeding. However, some fertility clinics use steroids on a short-term basis alongside IVF.
Antibiotics including penicillins, ampicillin, tetracyclines, erythromycin	Bacterial infections	Check with your GP if a particular prescribed antibiotic is safe in early pregnancy.
Antidepressants: selective serotonin re-uptake inhibitors (SSRIs) such as *Prozac*	Depression and anxiety	These can reduce libido, cause menstrual or ovulatory irregularities, and dry up or reduce cervical secretions. Discuss any risks or downsides relating to the drug with your GP or specialist so that you can decide whether to continue with a particular treatment.
Antispasmodics such as atropine, belladonna, dicyclomine, propantheline	Epilepsy	These can decrease cervical secretions, and/or cause thickening or dryness. Nutritional effect: they can lead to folic acid deficiency. Since all women trying to get pregnant should be taking a folic acid supplement (see page 105), you need to discuss with your GP how much you should be taking in addition to the recommended dose.
Antimalarial drugs such as mefloquine, atovaquone, and *Malarone* (proguanil), and tetracyclines	Malaria	Seek specialist advice on all antimalarial drugs. You may also need to take increased amounts of folic acid.
Methotrexate	Rheumatoid arthritis	Can cause birth defects. Nutritional effect: can cause folic acid deficiency, so supplements should be taken before pregnancy.

Q Have you ever had a miscarriage?

A miscarriage – defined as the loss of a pregnancy during the first 24 weeks' gestation – is a common problem. Around 15 per cent of confirmed pregnancies end in miscarriage; in 98 per cent of cases, this will occur in the first 12 weeks and will be the result of a random cause, which is unlikely to occur again. After one miscarriage, your chances of having a successful pregnancy are still 80 per cent, which is not much lower than if you have never been pregnant before.

That said, miscarriage rates do increase sharply with age and if you are over 35, you may wish to ask your doctor for tests if you miscarry for the first time (usually doctors will only refer you for tests after a third miscarriage). In this way, you can eliminate any underlying causes such as an autoimmune problem or adhesions (scar tissue) due to surgery or infection.

Losing a baby in this way is often mentally devastating. You may need professional support and counselling in order to help you deal with the psychological side of your pregnancy loss and help you to conceive again. A healthy diet and lifestyle, together with complementary therapies such as acupuncture, relaxation techniques, and yoga will ensure you are in the best possible physical and mental condition for a future pregnancy (see Steps 6 and 8).

Only 1 per cent of couples suffer recurrent miscarriage, which is defined as three or more consecutive pregnancy losses. If you are unlucky enough to be in this situation, it is best to get a referral to a specialist recurrent miscarriage unit at a hospital, where highly experienced staff will do the necessary tests to find out if there is something wrong, and will also treat you with the tender loving care which you no doubt need by now. Studies have shown that just by putting yourself in the care of the experts – even if they find nothing wrong with you – significantly raises the chances of a successful pregnancy outcome.

Q Have you had an ectopic pregnancy?

Around 1 in every 200 pregnancies ends in an ectopic pregnancy, which is when the embryo develops outside the uterine cavity. In almost all cases, it implants in one of the fallopian tubes. Initially, a woman will "feel" pregnant and a pregnancy test will be positive, although in many instances she may not even realize she is pregnant by the time the ectopic pregnancy causes problems.

ectopic pregnancy risk increases:

- if you have had previous abdominal surgery, particularly to the ovaries or fallopian tubes
- if you have undergone IVF treatment
- if you are aged between 35 and 44
- if you have previously had a pelvic infection such as chlamydia
- if you have had a previous ectopic pregnancy (one study found the likelihood increased by 50 to 80 per cent)

Symptoms include lower abdominal pain, which usually becomes severe and may be accompanied soon after by vaginal bleeding. Ectopic pregnancy can cause tubal damage if the fertilized egg stretches and bursts the fallopian tube as it attempts to grow. The damage may be irreversible.

Treatment usually involves surgery, although many hospitals are able to remove the pregnancy using laparoscopy, in which a fine tube with a camera on the end is inserted into the abdomen through a small incision, rather than more invasive surgery. Further tests will then be required to see if the damaged fallopian tube is still functioning adequately. It may be possible to treat certain early ectopic pregnancies non-surgically, by administering a methotrexate injection, which causes reabsorption of the pregnancy tissue.

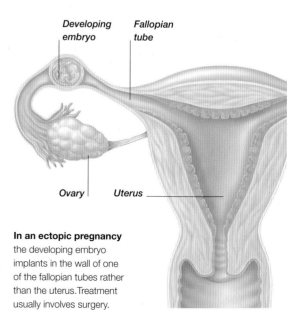

Developing embryo   *Fallopian tube*

Ovary   *Uterus*

In an ectopic pregnancy the developing embryo implants in the wall of one of the fallopian tubes rather than the uterus. Treatment usually involves surgery.

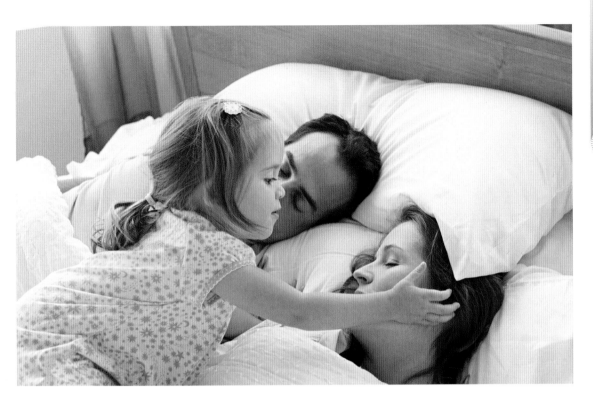

"Secondary infertility" may be simply due to the fact that the first baby or toddler is often in the parental bed.

If, following treatment for an ectopic pregnancy, one of your fallopian tubes suffers irreversible damage, your chances of conceiving naturally will be reduced. However, provided the remaining fallopian tube is healthy and has full mobility, it can sweep up an egg from the opposite, blocked tube. So, although the risk of a further ectopic pregnancy is increased, with careful early monitoring and scanning, women who conceive following an ectopic pregnancy have every chance of a successful outcome to their next pregnancy.

Q Can couples have problems conceiving if they already have children?

Sometimes, despite having had one or more children, a man or a woman can suffer from what is known as "secondary infertility". Often, it is because a new factor has arisen since that person's child or children were conceived that makes it difficult for pregnancy to happen. It may be an age-related problem (see pages 16–17) or it

may be that a couple are in a new relationship and there are children from previous relationships or financial worries that are causing tension and reducing the chances of conceiving. It could even be, quite simply, that there is a toddler who is still sleeping in the parental bed so sex happens much less frequently.

Alternatively, it may be that one partner has developed a medical condition that has affected his or her fertility, such as an underactive thyroid (see page 20), or that trauma following a previous birth is having an impact. Secondary infertility can be caused by a mixture of all these and other reasons (see also Step 3 on male infertility).

All forms of infertility can be extremely upsetting and frustrating and secondary infertility is no exception. Couples are left perplexed and confused about why this should be happening to them, and feel unable to move forward if their plans are centred on adding to their family. They may also find that friends and family are not as sympathetic as they might be.

Even if only one of you already has a child or children, you should both be investigated for infertility and together make any dietary and lifestyle changes that can maximize your chances of conceiving.

questionnaire: **a health check**

Answer these questions with your partner to help establish your **basic fertility** health as a couple. This is your **starting point** for deciding what **measures** to take as you make plans to conceive

1 Are you over 35 or is your partner (male) over 45?
yes ☐ **no** ☐
Age is a key determining factor in both female and male fertility.

2 Have you been trying to get pregnant for more than one year?
yes ☐ **no** ☐
Whatever your age, don't wait too long before seeking help. If you are in the age bracket of question 1, and have been trying for six months and having frequent sex, it's time to get help now.

3 Are you under- or overweight?
yes ☐ **no** ☐
A BMI of under 20 or over 25 could be impacting on your chances of conceiving. See page 13 and Step 6 for how to make sure weight is not a factor in your fertility.

4 Have you recently used the pill, an IUD, or a contraception injection or implant?
yes ☐ **no** ☐
These methods of contraception can affect your cervical secretions and your body's hormonal balance (see page 15).

5 Was your last smear test more than three years ago?
yes ☐ **no** ☐
There may be cell changes since your last test, which would need to be dealt with before you get pregnant. So make sure now that everything is OK.

6 Have you or your partner ever contracted an STI?
yes ☐ **no** ☐
These can affect fertility, particularly if left untreated. See pages 18–19.

7 Have you ever suffered or could you be suffering from fibroids, pelvic inflammatory disease, polycystic ovary syndrome, or endometriosis?
yes ☐ **no** ☐
These are all common causes of infertility, so check the symptoms on pages 22–23 and consult your doctor.

8 Do you suffer from thyroid disease, lupus, anaemia, or rheumatoid arthritis?
yes ☐ **no** ☐
These disorders can affect conception rates and/or increase the risk of a miscarriage. Check the symptoms on pages 20–21.

9 Do you suffer from any other long-term medical condition which could affect your fertility?
yes ☐ **no** ☐
Speak to your doctor to see if this could affect your chances of getting pregnant.

10 Are you regularly taking over-the-counter medication such as ibuprofen or antihistamines?
yes ☐ **no** ☐
Some medication can impact on fertility. Consult the chart on page 24 and talk to your doctor, if necessary.

11

Are you on prescribed medication?
yes ☐ **no** ☐
Don't stop taking a prescribed drug, but discuss your plans to get pregnant with your doctor to see if your treatment needs to be amended in any way.

12

Have you or your partner ever had chemotherapy or received radiotherapy to your abdomen?
yes ☐ **no** ☐
Speak to a specialist to find out if your fertility has been damaged (see page 14).

13

Do you or your partner have diabetes and struggle to control it?
yes ☐ **no** ☐
Although well-controlled diabetes doesn't affect fertility, high glucose levels do.

14

Did your mother go through a premature menopause?
yes ☐ **no** ☐
This condition is often hereditary so bear it in mind when planning to get pregnant.

15

Have you ever had abdominal surgery?
yes ☐ **no** ☐
Scar tissue can cause adhesions in the abdominal cavity and affect fertility.

16

Have you had more than three miscarriages?
yes ☐ **no** ☐
Unless you have had more than three successive miscarriages (see page 26) a one-off miscarriage should not be an indicator of reduced fertility.

17

Have you ever had an ectopic pregnancy?
yes ☐ **no** ☐
You may need to undergo tests to check for fallopian tube damage. You also run a higher risk of another ectopic pregnancy.

your**score**

0 If you had no "yes" answers, then you have nothing much to worry about regarding possible medical causes of infertility.

1–4 There is every chance that there is nothing wrong with your fertility. It is possible, though, that one or more of your "yes" answers could nonetheless affect your chances of conception, so make sure you take seriously any possible areas of concern. In addition, if you are over 35 or you have been trying to conceive for over a year (despite having plenty of sex), it is worth consulting a specialist now, just to make sure there is nothing wrong.

5–9 This score indicates that your fertility could be affected by several factors. Discuss the findings with your GP and arrange to see a fertility expert.

10–14 You are probably already aware that your fertility is being affected by your health. Seek medical advice as soon as possible, and follow the diet and lifestyle changes suggested in the book.

15–17 You will need significant help in getting pregnant, and may already be seeking specialist help to improve your chances of conceiving. Don't despair. You should also adopt diet and lifestyle changes that can make a real difference to your fertility.

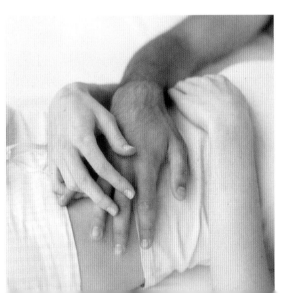

Gaining an understanding
of the way **female fertility**
works can be enough to solve
what appeared to be
a **fertility problem**

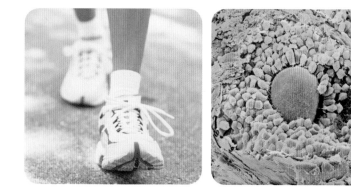
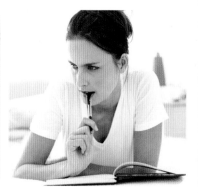

step**two**
basics for women

Your questions answered on:

step two: **basics for women**

This section is for **women's eyes only!** In it I cover all the key information about female fertility, so that you have as many facts as possible at your fingertips. These include **what happens** during the **menstrual cycle**, recognizing when you are at your **most fertile**, and understanding **how age can affect** your ability to conceive

Q What is considered to be a "normal" menstrual cycle?

Your menstrual cycle begins on day 1 of your period and lasts until the day before your next period. A mature egg is released (ovulation) mid cycle each month, usually around day 14 (see pages 36–37). A 28-day figure is always used as a convenient average, but in reality the length of the cycle varies considerably from one woman to another. If yours is between 23 and 35 days long, then it is considered normal, as long as it is regular, with no more than seven days' variation each month. Most periods last three to five days, but as long as they are regularly of the same duration (or almost), the length of the actual period is not important.

Q Are irregular cycles a sign that there is a fertility problem?

A cycle would be considered irregular if there is more than a seven-day variation month on month. Irregular periods or periods that are very light when they do happen (one or two days of very light bleeding or spotting) may indicate that you are suffering from a hormonal imbalance.

If your periods are more than 35 days apart, if you have only between four and nine periods per year, and if they are irregular and unpredictable, you are suffering from a disorder called oligomenorrhoea. This does not necessarily mean that you will be unable to conceive, but it may be difficult to predict when you are at your most fertile using the normal methods (see page 39). Alternative methods include ovulation-predictor kits but they may not be suitable for all women. One way of

predicting ovulation is to undergo follicular tracking where the ovaries are scanned on a regular basis using an ultrasound machine to determine when you are approaching ovulation.

Oligomenorrhoea can often be caused by lifestyle factors including:
- stress
- poor nutrition
- over-exercising
- weight
- frequent travel.

Reducing stress, being fit but not exercising obsessively, and eating a balanced diet that provides you with all the nutrients you need (see Steps 5 and 6) will help your body to function at its best, including hormonally, so this should always be a key line of attack if you suffer from irregular periods. You should also consult your GP to make sure that any underlying medical problems, such as polycystic ovary syndrome (see page 22) or thyroid disease (see page 20), are not the primary cause of your oligomenorrhoea.

Q My periods are regularly less than 21 days apart. Is this a problem?

Very short cycles could be a problem. In some cases, ovulation will be occurring very early (for example around day 7) and there will not be enough time for the egg to reach full maturity before it is released. Other women may have a reduced interval from ovulation to the next period (the luteal phase). If this phase is less than 10 days long, there will not be enough time for a fertilized egg to implant. If your periods are close together, you should discuss this with your GP or fertility specialist.

find out more: **female anatomy**

The internal organs of the female reproductive system are all located in the lower third of the abdomen. The ovaries store and release eggs, which pass along the fallopian tubes into the uterus. The vagina connects the uterus to the outside of the body. The visible external organs are collectively known as the vulva and consist of the sexually sensitive clitoris surrounded by folds of skin called the labia, which protect the entrances to the vagina and urethra.

fascinating **facts**

- The fallopian tube is approximately the width of a human hair.
- During pregnancy the uterus increases in weight from around 50g (2oz) to around 1kg (40oz).

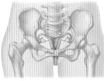

Location of uterus

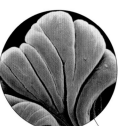

Fimbriae are finger-like projections that sweep eggs from the ovaries and guide them into the fallopian tubes.

The fallopian tube is lined with hair-like projections called cilia

The ovary contains egg follicles at different stages of development

The muscular wall of the uterus can stretch to accommodate a developing baby

The cervix is the neck of the uterus and projects into the vagina. Its central opening widens during childbirth

The endometrium (thickened lining of the uterus) looks spongy after ovulation and is ready to receive the fertilized egg.

Vagina

eggs developing in the ovary

Once a month, about 20 immature eggs start to develop within sacs in the ovaries known as follicles. Usually, only one egg will develop to full maturity while the others shrivel away. The primary follicle contains the egg which has grown the fastest. Once mature, the egg is about half the size of a grain of sand and is the largest cell in the human body.

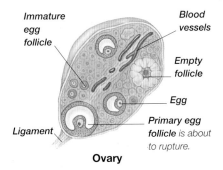

Immature egg follicle

Blood vessels

Empty follicle

Egg

Primary egg follicle is about to rupture.

Ligament

Ovary

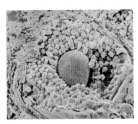

As the immature egg grows and develops, it absorbs nutrients from cells inside the follicle.

Q Can heavy periods be a symptom of infertility?

If you experience excessive bleeding that continues for several days and you also notice the passing of blood clots, this can be a sign that you suffer from what is called menorrhagia and you must consult your GP to try to find the cause of the problem. As a result of losing a lot of blood, you may also have become anaemic (see page 21) and feel permanently exhausted, so your doctor should arrange for a blood test to be done to check your iron levels. Menorrhagia can also be caused by:

■ endometriosis
■ pelvic inflammatory disease
■ fibroids
■ thyroid disease.

These conditions are common causes of infertility (see pages 18–19 and 22) and require conventional treatment.

Whatever the reason for menorrhagia, good nutrition, regular exercise, and certain complementary therapies, such as acupuncture, can help to alleviate the symptoms (see Steps 5, 6, and 8).

Q Is mid-cycle spotting or bleeding something to worry about?

Yes, it may be, as it is not usually normal to have bleeding between periods. This may have a variety of causes, including uterine fibroids, polyps, infections and, occasionally, cervical cancer. Consequently, any such bleeding should be reported to your doctor. It is also very important to make sure that your smear test is up to date. Your GP may suggest rechecking your smear, and may also take swabs to check for infections. Further investigations may then be required to find the reason for the bleeding. If, after further tests, no cause can be found, then for some women, light bleeding or spotting is a normal occurrence and may be linked to fluctuating oestrogen/progesterone levels around the time of ovulation. This should not impact on your ability to conceive and can be a sign of a highly fertile time in your cycle.

Q What sort of sanitary protection is it best to use?

I'm not a great advocate of tampons even though the jury is out on whether they have an impact on fertility: one study conducted with over 2,000 women concluded

that women who used tampons had a lower rate of endometriosis (see page 22) than those who did not, the theory being that tampons suck out debris rather than push it back into the uterus. However, others believe that tampons encourage a retrograde menstrual flow.

If you do want to use tampons, choose unbleached, 100 per cent cotton ones that allow free flow, and restrict their use to the times when the flow is heavy and the tampon is soaked through. Change them frequently to avoid any risk of developing the rare but serious toxic shock syndrome, caused when bacterial growth occurs in the vagina, and toxins are released into the bloodstream. Symptoms include a high fever, a rash, and low blood pressure.

On days when the flow is lighter use pads because tampons tend to absorb the vagina's protective secretions and moisture too. For the same reason women who are pre-disposed to vaginal dryness, thrush, or cystitis are better off using pads. I would also suggest you use pads at night.

Q I'm not pregnant, but I haven't had a period for six months. Why?

If a woman does not have a period at all for six months, this is called amenorrhoea and is a clear indication that there is a hormonal problem because ovulation has in effect ceased. If this happens to you, you must always see your GP. However, in practice, you should not wait for six months but instead consult your doctor if, at any time, your cycle changes in nature or you develop an unusual delay between your periods.

Amenorrhoea can be caused by several factors, including:
■ a hormonal problem involving the pituitary, thyroid, or adrenal glands
■ having been on the pill or using contraceptive injections.
■ severe stress
■ extreme weight loss or having a BMI below 18.5 (see page 13)
■ an eating disorder
■ an ovarian problem such as premature menopause
■ excessive exercise.

You may need some hormone treatment to enable your body to start ovulating again. It may also be that by changing a particular aspect of your lifestyle and/or diet, you can restore your hormonal balance and start ovulating again. However, in the first instance, before assuming that the disruption in your cycle is down to lifestyle causes, I would always advise women to seek medical advice.

find out more: **painful periods**

The medical term used to describe painful periods (including severe menstrual cramps) is dysmenorrhoea. Painful periods are more likely to occur when a woman's cycle is irregular and can be extremely uncomfortable, with severe pain felt in the lower back, abdomen, and inner thighs. This may be particularly so if the menstrual cycle has been very long, as there has been more time for the hormone progesterone to cause the build-up of a thicker womb lining. Painful periods can also be caused by underlying conditions such as endometriosis or fibroids (see pages 22–23).

Up to 60 per cent of women suffer from menstrual cramps, and some end up doing so in silence for years without realizing that they actually have a medical condition that affects their ability to conceive. If your periods are very painful, you should see your GP to arrange for specialist tests to be done rather than accepting the pain as normal and resorting to the use of painkillers.

watch your **medication**

Some women I come across are frequent users of painkillers such as ibuprofen and aspirin. Yet, excessive use of these drugs, particularly ibuprofen, can have a harmful effect on their fertility (see page 24). If you need to take a painkiller for menstrual cramps, try to manage with paracetamol.

taking a natural approach

Painful periods may be made worse by lifestyle factors (see page 32). If this is the case there are steps you can take to help manage the symptoms.

■ Take gentle, endorphin-releasing exercise (such as swimming, walking, or cycling) during the painful day(s). Endorphins act as the body's natural painkillers.

■ Learn relaxation techniques to reduce the levels of tension in your body. Tension exacerbates pain.

■ Apply heat to your abdomen. Simple steps, such as applying a hot water bottle, microwave-heated cushion, or small heat pad to the abdomen, are very helpful.

■ TENS machines, which use electrical impulses to block pain signals, can help to alleviate the pain.

■ Try acupuncture. Research has shown that it can help reduce the levels of pain and the need for medication in women suffering from dysmenorrhoea. Acupuncture pads are now available.

■ Some women find that good nutrition helps reduce the level of period pain they experience. Make sure you are eating foods that are rich in magnesium, vitamin E and vitamin B1 or try taking supplements that include these (see pages 104–106).

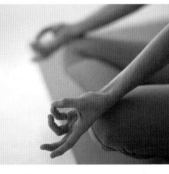

Exercise triggers the release of the body's natural pain-relieving endorphins.

Relaxation techniques such as yoga help reduce tension, which can exacerbate pain.

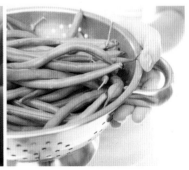

Eating foods, such as green beans, that have key nutrients may help painful periods.

find out more: **the female cycle**

If you are trying to get pregnant, it helps to **understand fully** your menstrual cycle so that you know when you are **at your most fertile**.

Although the average cycle lasts for 28 days, there is considerable variation among women and it is considered perfectly normal to have cycles that are longer or shorter than this. That said, even if your cycle falls within what is considered to be the normal range, you might not be producing the right level of a particular hormone at the right time to trigger ovulation and provide the right conditions for a fertilized egg to implant, and this could be enough to prevent you from getting pregnant.

calculating **fertility**

Note the length of six cycles. Take your shortest cycle and subtract 20; then your longest and subtract 10. If the results were, for example, 6 and 21 then you are potentially fertile between days 6 and 21.

the menstrual cycle

The female cycle is driven by a complex interaction of hormones that need to be secreted at the correct level for fertility. The cycle is divided into two phases: the follicular phase, which lasts from day 1 of your period until ovulation; and the luteal phase, which lasts from ovulation until the start of your next period.

the follicular phase On day 1 of the menstrual cycle, the hypothalamus (often referred to as the control centre in the brain) secretes gonadotrophin-releasing hormone (GnRH). This tells the pituitary gland, situated deep inside the brain, to produce follicle-stimulating hormone (FSH). Over the next couple of weeks, the levels of FSH in the bloodstream rise and enable sac-like follicles in the ovaries to grow. Each follicle contains an egg and although around 20 eggs start to ripen each month, only one (or occasionally two) will become fully mature. The others

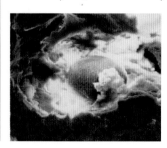

At ovulation, the egg follicle bursts and the mature egg inside it is released.

will gradually shrivel up and disappear. Each egg is surrounded by granulosa cells, which feed it and also produce oestrogen. Oestrogen has many roles during the follicular phase:

- Rising levels of oestrogen tell the pituitary gland to reduce the production of FSH so that, usually, only one egg is released at ovulation.
- Oestrogen starts to thicken the lining of the uterus (the endometrium) in preparation for implantation of an embryo, should fertilization of the egg occur. Oestrogen opens up the cervix and thins the cervical secretions, assisting the passage of sperm.
- Oestrogen tells the hypothalamus that the follicle is mature; the hypothalamus then sends a message back to the pituitary gland to produce a short burst, or pulse, of luteinising hormone (LH). This enables the follicle to burst, usually 24 to 36 hours later, and the fully mature egg inside it to be released. This is known as ovulation.

Ovulation takes place from one ovary only, although there is no evidence to indicate that it occurs on alternate sides from one month to the next.

The follicular phase can be quite varied in length. It typically lasts around 14 days but it will be shorter or longer depending on the length of your cycle and on whether or not your cycles are irregular.

the luteal phase Post ovulation, the ruptured follicle continues to receive pulses of LH as it turns into a small cyst-like swelling called the corpus luteum that starts to produce progesterone, which has several effects:

- It thickens the endometrium.
- It produces the nutrients that maintain a pregnancy until the placenta can take over.
- It switches off secretion of FSH and LH.
- It closes the cervix and thickens the cervical secretions, preventing passage of sperm.
- It raises body temperature by approximately 0.2°C, thus preparing the uterus for a fertilized egg.

After ovulation, the finger-like projections at the end of the fallopian tube pick up the egg. The tube is lined with

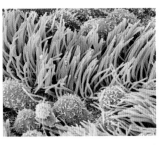

Microscopic hairs line the fallopian tubes, helping to propel the egg along.

microscopic hairs, called cilia, which, along with muscular contractions, propel the egg towards the uterus. If the egg is not fertilized along the way, it gradually disintegrates. Oestrogen and progesterone levels fall until the lining of the uterus cannot be maintained, and menstruation begins.

changes during the menstrual cycle

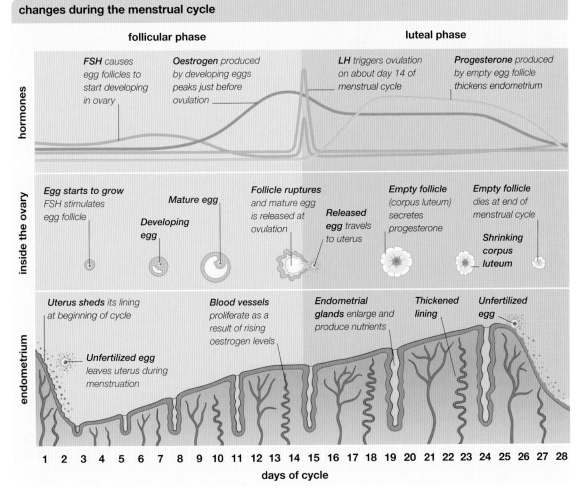

follicular phase

luteal phase

hormones

FSH causes egg follicles to start developing in ovary

Oestrogen produced by developing eggs peaks just before ovulation

LH triggers ovulation on about day 14 of menstrual cycle

Progesterone produced by empty egg follicle thickens endometrium

inside the ovary

Egg starts to grow
FSH stimulates egg follicle

Developing egg

Mature egg

Follicle ruptures and mature egg is released at ovulation

Released egg travels to uterus

Empty follicle (corpus luteum) secretes progesterone

Empty follicle dies at end of menstrual cycle

Shrinking corpus luteum

endometrium

Uterus sheds its lining at beginning of cycle

Unfertilized egg leaves uterus during menstruation

Blood vessels proliferate as a result of rising oestrogen levels

Endometrial glands enlarge and produce nutrients

Thickened lining

Unfertilized egg

1 2 3 4 5 6 7 8 9 10 11 12 13 14 15 16 17 18 19 20 21 22 23 24 25 26 27 28

days of cycle

Q How does age affect ovulation?

Hormonal changes start to take place as you move towards the pre-menopausal years and these affect your menstrual cycle and fertility. If you are over 35, as well as a reduction in the number and quality of your eggs and the risks and complications that this entails (see page 16), you sometimes release two mature eggs at ovulation, rather than the usual one. This explains the higher incidence of non-identical twins among women over the age of 35.

In addition, your cycle often starts to become shorter and/or less regular. Consequently, the day on which you ovulate can fluctuate, making it more difficult to know when you are fertile. Your cervical mucus may be drier because you are secreting less oestrogen.

Q What is a luteal phase defect?

This is an ovulation disorder where an egg is released but the corpus luteum (the yellow structure left in the ovary after ovulation) does not produce enough progesterone. As a result, the lining of the uterus does not thicken properly and a fertilized egg is unable to embed. The luteal phase (the time from ovulation to the next period or post-ovulation phase, see page 37) is often shorter than it should be.

Sometimes treatment may be given in the form of clomiphene: this is an ovulation stimulation drug, which in effect boosts ovulation and thereby increases the progesterone level, maintaining the thicker lining of the uterus to give enough time for the fertilized egg to implant. If this is not effective, then assisted conception such as IVF may be used.

Q How can I tell if I am approaching the menopause?

Signs of the menopause include a regular menstrual cycle becoming increasingly irregular, hot flushes, night sweats, mood swings, and vaginal dryness. It is important to be aware of these when you are planning a pregnancy, particularly if your mother experienced early menopause (before the age of 40), as this condition may be hereditary (see page 14).

Most women are perimenopausal up to 10 years before their periods stop altogether. If you suspect you may be approaching the menopause yet are hoping to become pregnant you should talk to your GP about having tests done to measure levels of AMH (anti-mullerian hormone), which goes down just before the menopause, and FSH, which goes up (see page 12). These will help to provide some indication of your current level of fertility.

Q How would I know if there was something wrong with my cycle?

There are various indicators that there might be something amiss with your menstrual cycle. These include a sudden lack of periods (especially if you have just come off the pill), a change in the regularity of your periods with lots of fluctuations from one month to the next, or if you start to experience a lot of pain.

If anything changes in your cycle, you should talk to your GP who will probably arrange for tests to be carried out. These will include a full blood test, as well as individual blood tests at different points during your cycle measuring levels of FSH, LH, thyroxine, and progesterone (see pages 141–142 for further details).

Another problem indicator to get checked out immediately is any spotting during your cycle (see page 34), as in some cases this could indicate cervical cancer.

Q Should I monitor whether or not I am ovulating each month?

As a rise in temperature each month shows that you have ovulated (see opposite page), you could try monitoring this for one month to check. However, although once is fine, at my clinic we dissuade women from taking their temperature month after month as a means of monitoring ovulation as it can make them very obsessive. I sometimes see women worrying over a year's worth of charts. Temperatures vary enormously with lots of factors, including lack of sleep, flu, or alcohol intake.

Using an ovulation kit (see opposite page) is a good way of learning to recognize when you ovulate, but this should only be done in combination with an understanding of your cervical secretions which vary throughout the menstrual cycle and are a guide to your fertile time (see page 40). The only wholly reliable way to check that ovulation is taking place is by having a blood test to check progesterone or an ultrasound scan, which your doctor would need to arrange.

Q How can I tell when **I am fertile**?

There are several ways in which you can recognize your fertile time and signs of approaching ovulation, and the more familiar you are with your menstrual cycle, the easier it will be. If you are in any doubt, a specially trained fertility awareness nurse at a family planning clinic can help you.

LH surge This is measured by ovulation-predictor kits that are now sold in pharmacies. However, if you wait to see the magic line on the pee stick before having sex, you will be very close to ovulation and may not have allowed sufficient time for the sperm to get to the egg and fertilize it. The test can also produce a false-positive in women who suffer from hormonal problems such as PCOS.

Basal body temperature (BBT) Progesterone causes body temperature to rise by about 0.2°C (0.4°F) immediately after ovulation and to stay at that level until your next period begins. Temperature can be a useful way of confirming that ovulation is occurring for some women, but by the time the temperature rises, ovulation will have happened, so this sign is really of no help in timing sex to get pregnant. Also, there are other factors that can affect temperature, such as a late night or stress.

Cervical secretions (see page 40) These are the most useful way of determining when you are fertile. Their appearance and consistency varies during your cycle and familiarizing yourself with these changes is essential if you are to maximize your chances of conceiving.

changes during the menstrual cycle

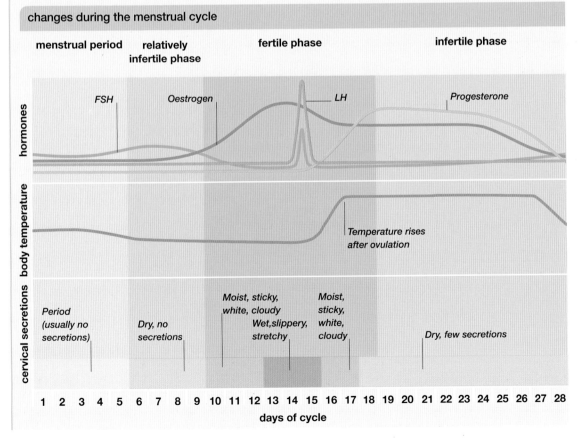

| menstrual period | relatively infertile phase | | fertile phase | | infertile phase |

hormones

FSH   Oestrogen   LH   Progesterone

body temperature

Temperature rises after ovulation

cervical secretions

Period (usually no secretions)   Dry, no secretions   Moist, sticky, white, cloudy / Wet, slippery, stretchy   Moist, sticky, white, cloudy   Dry, few secretions

1 2 3 4 5 6 7 8 9 10 11 12 13 14 15 16 17 18 19 20 21 22 23 24 25 26 27 28

days of cycle

Q What part do cervical secretions play in fertility?

The quantity and consistency of the mucus secreted from the cervix varies considerably during the menstrual cycle. During the optimum conditions for conception, the secretions nourish the sperm and help them to swim towards the egg. The changes are due to hormonal fluctuations, and, although it might take you a little while to learn to recognize these differences, you will benefit afterwards from knowing when you are at your most fertile. Aim to note down the variations in your secretions over the course of a few cycles, until you feel familiar with their changes in appearance. Based on a 28-day cycle, the pattern of secretions will be similar to the one shown below.

If you are taking the pill, there may be changes in your secretions. Remember that when you come off the pill it may be a few months before everything returns to normal.

Q How are cervical secretions affected by longer or shorter cycles?

You will need to calculate, based on observation over the course of three to four cycles, when and how your mucus changes. You may find, if your cycle is short, that you actually ovulate a few days after the end of your period and so will notice fertile cervical secretions towards the end of your period. If this is the case, then this will be the best time for sex to optimize your chances of conception. Conversely, if your cycle is 35 days long, ovulation could be taking place around day 21.

Q Why am I finding it difficult to work out when my cervical secretions are "fertile"?

There are a variety of reasons why your cervical secretions might not follow a regular pattern or appearance. These include:

cervical secretions and fertility		
days	type of secretions	fertile?
1–5	Menstrual blood.	No (unless your cycle is very short)
7–9	Dry. No secretions seen or felt.	Relatively infertile
10–12	Moist and sticky feel, white or cloudy appearance. Oestrogen levels increasing. If you try to stretch mucus between your thumb and forefinger, it will break.	Yes
13–15	Wet and slippery feel, clear appearance, like raw egg white. Caused by high oestrogen levels. If testing the mucus between the thumb and forefinger, it will stretch rather than break. Intercourse at the time you notice these secretions gives the highest chance of pregnancy.	Highly fertile time
16–17	Moist and sticky feel, white or cloudy appearance (although some women will change to dryness, rather than moist and sticky secretions). If you try to stretch the mucus between your thumb and forefinger it will break. The peak day is the last day of the wetter secretions and is recognized retrospectively because the following day will be either dry or moist and sticky. The thicker secretions, caused by a rise in progesterone and fall in oestrogen, form a plug at the cervix, which may block the sperm and prevent them from getting any further.	Fertile for three days after the peak day
18–28	Dry. No or few secretions seen or felt.	No

- You may be ovulating at the end of your period, particularly if your cycle is short.
- Your oestrogen levels may be low, perhaps because you have a low BMI or exercise excessively.
- You may be using medication (prescription or over-the-counter) that affects your mucus, making it drier or thicker than it should be.
- Your periods are irregular or infrequent, making it difficult to detect when you are at your most fertile.
- You may recently have come off the pill and your cycle may not have had time to return to normal (see page 15).

A fertility awareness consultant should be able to help.

Q Is the missionary position better for conceiving than other positions?

There is no evidence to suggest that this is the case. That said, many couples use different positions during sex but choose to finish with the woman underneath. Whatever you decide, you may prefer to stay lying down for 20 to 30 minutes afterwards, just to give the sperm a bit of a start in their journey through the cervix and into the uterus. Even if you are not underneath your partner when he ejaculates, and even if you do lose seminal fluid because you move around after intercourse, you can be sure that, provided you are having sex at a fertile time of your cycle, the position you are in should not make any difference to whether you can conceive. Millions of sperm are released in every ejaculate (see page 51), so losing a few will not make any difference!

Q Does having an orgasm help a woman to conceive?

It probably helps to be aroused and therefore well lubricated during intercourse as a wetter vagina will help the sperm to swim. Having an orgasm may also facilitate the sperm's journey thanks to the vaginal spasms that occur. However, fortunately, achieving orgasm is absolutely not necessary to become pregnant. What is more important (and the same applies to the question of whether you should be underneath when your partner ejaculates) is staying relaxed, not letting sex become "baby sex" (see Step 4) and maintaining a good sexual relationship with your partner.

case**study**

Sarah and Bob had been trying to conceive for almost a year when they decided to seek advice on fertility and fertile times from a specialist.

Sarah When Bob and I decided to start trying for a baby I always made sure we had plenty of sex between days 10 and 16 of my cycle, based on the fact that I thought that ovulation occurs on day 14. When nothing happened I decided to go and see a fertility awareness specialist and in doing so I discovered a lot of information about my menstrual cycle and fertility that I had never been aware of in the past.

The specialist explained to me that because my cycles vary in length, lasting between 25 days and 36 days, these would be considered irregular and as a result, the day on which I ovulate varies from one month to the next: in some cycles it would be early and in other cycles it would be much later. In order to get a better idea as to when I am fertile, the specialist then taught me how to monitor the cyclical changes in my cervical secretions and I started to look out for the secretions that would indicate my fertile time.

On my next period, as my period was getting light, I noticed some clear, slippery secretions mixed with the light bleeding. So, we broke away from our usual pattern and had sex. We were delighted the next month when my period never came and a pregnancy test proved positive. We had conceived from having sex on day 6 of my cycle!

This confirms the fact that having sex only around day 14 could, in some instances, be the reason for not getting pregnant rather than any more complicated fertility issue.

Q Is it best to have sex only on the day of ovulation?

Healthy sperm can live in the female reproductive tract for several days, but the ripe ovum needs to be fertilized within 24 hours of ovulation. This means that you can conceive after having had sex several days before ovulation, but once you have ovulated, you have only about 24 hours in which to have sexual intercourse that can lead to a conception.

Although there are useful indications, it is almost impossible to predict the precise day of ovulation without the help of an ultrasound scan. Experts now agree that, to maximize the chances of conception, couples should have sex frequently from the time a woman first notices any cervical secretions (usually sticky white secretions), through the time of any clearer, wetter secretions, and for three days after the secretions change back to either sticky white or dryness again (see page 40). Ideally, this means having sex every two to three days and daily for the two to three days around the time of the wetter secretions.

Abstinence can also harm sperm function, although sperm can live for up to seven days in the female reproductive tract; one study found that 94 per cent of pregnancies were attributed to sperm that were one or two days old.

Q How long can I afford to wait before I start trying to get pregnant?

Although all experts agree that female fertility starts to decline sharply once a woman gets beyond the age of 35, there is also no disputing the fact that more and more women are having babies late in their reproductive life. And although I would like to remind women not to play Russian roulette too much with their fertility, I also want to emphasise that many women are able to produce healthy babies until well into their 40s.

The window of opportunity for getting pregnant is wide (about six days), although the chance of conception on each of the six days for a woman in her late 30s will be only about half that of a woman in her early 20s. I believe that the more you give yourself the best chance of conceiving, by understanding your body and how it works, adopting a healthy lifestyle, staying as relaxed as possible – and having a lot of sex – the higher your chance of conception (see pages 16–17).

find out more: conception

During sexual arousal, the man's penis becomes erect and the woman's vagina is lubricated. During intercourse, the penis is inserted into the vagina and the man begins thrusting pelvic movements. At orgasm, the man ejaculates and releases sperm. These then begin their long journey to the egg.

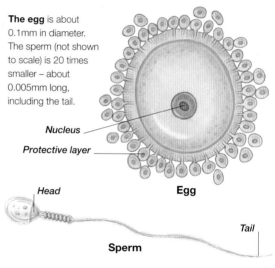

The egg is about 0.1mm in diameter. The sperm (not shown to scale) is 20 times smaller – about 0.005mm long, including the tail.

Nucleus

Protective layer

Head

Egg

Tail

Sperm

two cells become one

Once a sperm reaches the egg and succeeds in breaching its shell, the sperm's head (the part containing the genetic information) enters and its tail is shed. A membrane then forms around the egg, creating a barrier to prevent other sperm from entering. Fertilization occurs when the head of the sperm fuses with the nucleus of the egg.

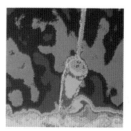

When fertilization occurs, many sperm swarm around the ripe egg, but only one manages to penetrate the outer shell and fuse with the nucleus.

from egg to embryo

Pregnancy begins when an egg is fertilized by a sperm, usually in the fallopian tube. Within two days of fertilization, the egg starts its journey towards the uterus, propelled by the muscular action of the fallopian tube. As the egg travels, its cells gradually divide to form a cluster of cells called a morula. At each stage the dividing cells become smaller, gradually reaching normal body cell size. After 3 to 4 days, the morula arrives in the uterus and develops a fluid-filled cavity and an inner cell mass. The morula is now known as a blastocyst. The blastocyst floats within the uterus for around 48 hours before landing on the thick uterine lining (endometrium), which softens to help implantation.

Within the blastocyst's inner cell mass, a two-layered disc forms. The top layer becomes the embryo and the amniotic cavity; the lower layer becomes the yolk sac, which helps to transport nutrients to the embryo during the second and third weeks. The amniotic cavity develops into a sac that fills with fluid and folds around the embryo and the yolk sac. The disc develops three circular sheets from which all the body structures will derive.

fascinating facts

- Of all the different types of cell in the body, the egg cell is the only spherical one.
- Morula is the Latin name for "mulberry" – the cell cluster is shaped like the fruit.

A two-cell embryo forms within 24–36 hours as the fertilized egg divides on it journey along the fallopian tube.

The embryo continues to divide several times to form a solid cluster of 16–32 cells called a morula. Around 3–4 days after fertilization, this enters the uterus.

Fallopian tube

The egg is fertilized by a single sperm in the fallopian tube – at this stage it consists of a single cell.

Ovary

About 5–6 days after fertilization, the cell cluster forms a hollow cavity and is known as a blastocyst. This then lands on the thick uterine lining and implants.

Uterus

Vagina

questionnaire: **is your cycle causing you problems?**

Using what you have read in this section, answer the questions here to find out **if your menstrual cycle is abnormal** in any way or if changes occur from one month to the next. By scoring 1 for each "yes", you will **gain some insight** into whether or not there are problems that could be **affecting your chance of conceiving**

1 Are your periods more than 35 days apart and/or irregular and unpredictable?
yes ☐ **no** ☐
You could have oligomenorrhoea (see page 32) and this will make it difficult for you to know when you are ovulating.

2 Do you find that the length of your menstrual cycle varies when you are under stress?
yes ☐ **no** ☐
If stress is causing irregularities in your cycle, it may be affecting your ovulation and therefore your fertility. You need to address lifestyle issues (see Step 5).

3 Have your periods ever ceased for several months?
yes ☐ **no** ☐
This is called amenorrhoea (see page 34) and you should consult a doctor to try to find the cause of this lack of ovulation.

4 Are your periods very close together?
yes ☐ **no** ☐
If your cycles are shorter than 23 days you may have problems with ovulation and implantation (see page 32).

5 Do you suffer from unusually heavy periods?
yes ☐ **no** ☐
This is called menorrhagia (see page 34) and it could be impacting on your fertility, so you should consult your doctor to try to find the cause.

6 Do you have any mid-cycle spotting or bleeding?
yes ☐ **no** ☐
Any bleeding, however light, should be investigated to rule out the presence of a potentially serious condition.

7 Do you suffer from painful periods?
yes ☐ **no** ☐
This is called dysmenorrhoea (see page 35). Consult your doctor to discover the cause of the pain as this could be a symptom of a disorder that affects fertility.

8 Do you regularly take painkillers for period pain?
yes ☐ **no** ☐
Excessive use of some painkillers can affect ovulation (see page 24) and mask the cause of pain. It is important to know what is causing pain as this may also be affecting your fertility.

9 Are you having difficulty recognizing changes in your cervical secretions?
yes ☐ **no** ☐

Learning to recognize the differences in your secretions can help you to work out when you are at your most fertile (see page 40).

10 Do you abstain from sex until the time when you believe that you are likely to be ovulating?
yes ☐ **no** ☐

Couples who have sex frequently during the time when the woman is fertile have a higher chance of conceiving than those who abstain until ovulation (see page 42).

11 If you are over 35, has your menstrual cycle become shorter?
yes ☐ **no** ☐

As you get older ovulation occurs earlier and less frequently. This may be making your cycle less predictable (see page 38).

your**score**

0–3 Although you are experiencing few problems with your cycle, the information in this chapter may help you understand it more fully, so that you know when you are at your most fertile. Consult a doctor if any areas are giving you cause for concern.

4–6 You should see your GP to make sure that the problems you are having regarding your cycle are investigated fully because some of these may be affecting your chances of conceiving. Consider also whether your lifestyle and dietary habits could be contributing to these problems (see Steps 5–7).

7–11 You need to treat the causes of your menstrual cycle's problems as in all likelihood this will improve your fertility. Both conventional medical treatment and complementary therapies should be able to help (read Step 8 to find out which ones are most likely to help). Always make sure you have a proper medical check-up before turning to complementary therapies.

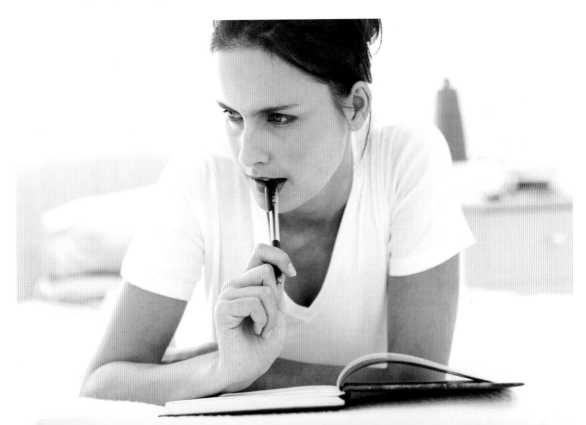

I meet many men who **understand very little** about their bodies and how they can **influence their potential** to become fathers

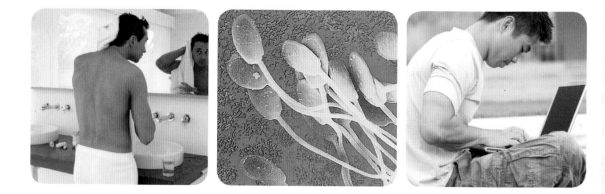

step**three**
basics for men

Your questions answered on:

step three: **basics for men**

Men are often **not very knowledgeable** about their own bodies and how they work, so this section aims to provide the information couples need **to understand male reproduction**. This step also highlights the main areas of **men's health** – aside from lifestyle factors such as alcohol and diet – which can have an impact on fertility

Q Is male fertility all about testosterone?

Levels of testosterone vary from one man to another but, assuming these are within a normal range, they are not linked to how fertile he might be. Indeed, it is very important for men to understand that any fertility problems they may have bear no relation whatsoever to their virility.

Men start to secrete sex hormones at puberty, which usually occurs between the ages of 12 and 14. As is the case with women, the hypothalamus in the brain acts as the control centre. It secretes gonadotrophin-releasing hormones and these cause the pituitary gland to produce follicle-stimulating hormone (FSH) and luteinizing hormone (LH). These in turn stimulate the testes to produce sperm. Luteinizing hormone also stimulates the testes to produce testosterone, which is responsible for the development of male secondary sex characteristics including facial and pubic hair, a deep voice, and increased muscle mass, all of which start at puberty.

Q Do men stop being fertile when they get older?

Like any cell in the body, sperm cells age, and the older we get, the more free radical damage there is to our cells and therefore to sperm cells as well. As I explained

Zita's **tip**

Men produce sperm **24 hours a day, every day**, so much can be done to improve sperm quality.

on page 17, age does start to affect a man's fertility: from the age of 35, he begins to produce a higher proportion of abnormal sperm (16 per cent in men over the age of 45, compared to 4 per cent for those in their late 20s). Maturing sperm must divide an estimated 380 times before they become adult sperm and, as the man ages, fewer cell divisions take place, leading to a higher number of abnormalities. As a result, although sperm production never ceases, there is a higher proportion of sperm which are abnormal-looking, unable to swim fast, or more likely to carry a genetic defect.

Furthermore, hormonal changes, poor blood supply to the testes, or impotence can also have an impact. Consequently, after the age of 50, most men will have some degree of testicular failure and, although their sperm production never ceases entirely, their ability to father a child will inevitably begin to decline.

Q Can a man have fertility problems if he has already fathered children?

If there has been more than a two-year gap since a man previously fathered a child, then yes, it is possible that he might no longer be as fertile as he was in the past. This is particularly the case if certain circumstances in his life have changed – if he is in a new relationship, for example. The onset of medical conditions such as diabetes can also affect fertility (see pages 52–53), and if a man is over the age of 45 he may find that his sperm quality and quantity have gone down.

So, although the ability to father a child in the past is an encouraging sign, it is not necessarily proof of a man's ongoing fertility.

find out more: **male anatomy**

The male genitals consist of the penis and scrotum, which contains two testes that produce sperm. Mature sperm move into a coiled tube behind each testis called an epididymis. Sperm are stored here before moving to another tube, the vas deferens. Each vas deferens connects an epididymis to an ejaculatory duct, which joins the urethra, the tube that passes along the penis. Sperm are carried in fluid produced by glands called seminal vesicles.

fascinating **facts**

- The epididymis is about 6m (18ft) long but only 0.76mm in diameter.
- The testes also contain Leydig cells, which manufacture the sex hormone testosterone.

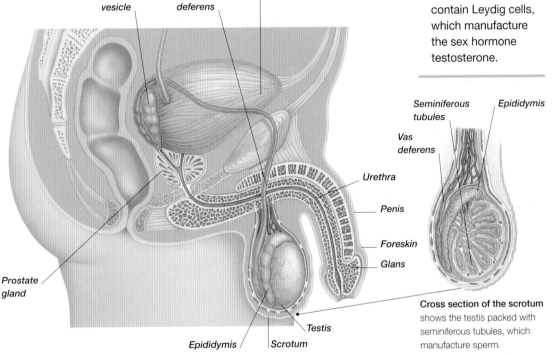

Seminal vesicle — Vas deferens — Bladder

Prostate gland

Epididymis — Scrotum — Testis

Urethra — Penis — Foreskin — Glans

Seminiferous tubules — Epididymis — Vas deferens

Cross section of the scrotum shows the testis packed with seminiferous tubules, which manufacture sperm.

how does an erection occur?

An erection begins with sensory and mental stimulation.

- The urethra, the tube down which both urine and ejaculate are expelled from the body, runs along the penis and is situated beneath two chambers called the *corpora cavernosa*, which are filled with veins, arteries, smooth muscle, and fibrous tissue.
- The urethra is surrounded by spongy tissue called the *corpus spongiosum*.
- When a man begins to be sexually aroused, impulses from his brain tell the muscles in the *corpora cavernosa* to relax, thereby enabling blood to flow into the tissues via the arteries.
- The additional blood causes pressure in the chambers, and as a result these expand and the penis becomes erect. A membrane surrounding the *corpora cavernosa*, called the *tunica albuginea*, then traps the blood and this allows the erection to be maintained.

Spongy tissue of the corpora cavernosum — Urethra — Artery

Section through the penis shows how it contains spongy tissue and blood vessels.

Q How long does sperm production take?

The production of mature sperm takes approximately 100 days, and in this time 380 cell divisions are required for the sperm to develop fully (compared with the 23 cell divisions required for an egg to reach maturity). Production begins in the seminiferous tubules in the testes, when FSH causes cell divisions in primary sperm cells, called spermatocytes. These develop into immature tail-less sperm called spermatids, and over the next 72 days cell division continues until the sperm are almost fully mature. The sperm then move into the epididymis and continues to mature for another 20 to 30 days, by which time they are ready to move up to the vas deferens, in preparation for ejaculation. It therefore takes around three months to notice any change to sperm quality or quantity.

Q What happens at ejaculation?

At ejaculation (orgasm), sperm are propelled from the epididymis and vas deferens into the urethra where they mix with secretions from the seminal vesicle and prostate, which lie just before the beginning of the urethra, just beneath the bladder. This combination forms the seminal fluid (or semen). Sperm only make up about 20 per cent of the volume; the rest is made up of more than 20 different chemical-like substances that help to nourish the sperm and enable them to survive the journey through the cervix and on through the female reproductive tract. The urethra is the passage out of the penis for both seminal fluid and urine, so a complex system of valves is required to make sure it is used for only one function at a time. When semen is ejaculated, it is viscous in consistency, but after about 10 minutes it begins to liquefy, to help the sperm to swim more easily through the cervical canal.

The vas deferens has a huge capacity and it may take around 30 ejaculations to empty the tube of its full load of sperm.

Q How much is a "normal" quantity of semen?

Approximately 2 to 4 millilitres of semen are produced per ejaculate, which is around half a teaspoonful. However, it is the quality of sperm that determines whether the man is fertile, not the quantity of semen he produces.

Q Tight underpants: fact or fiction when it comes to fertility?

There is no doubt that any increased or prolonged heat to the testes reduces semen count and quality. Research on taxi drivers (who sit for prolonged periods) and laptop users (see page 55) has confirmed this. Testicles need to be a few degrees below body temperature for optimum sperm function, which is why the scrotum is designed to hang more loosely away from the body in hot weather and pull in towards it in cold weather so that a steady temperature is maintained. Wearing tight underpants for prolonged periods could increase scrotal temperature. I advise men to go for comfort in terms of underpants – the lighter the better – and to avoid tight jeans.

Q Is it true that sperm determine the sex of a baby?

Yes, it is the sperm that determines the sex of a child. A woman's ovum and a man's sperm each carry a single set of 23 chromosomes. A unique mix of genes is spread over these 23 chromosomes, and when an egg is fertilized the embryo has 23 pairs of chromosomes, one set from each parent. Numbers 45 and 46 (pair 23) are the sex chromosomes, which determine the sex of the child. The mother's egg always carries the female chromosome (which is given the label X). The father's sperm, however, carries either the female chromosome, X, or the male one (labelled as Y). When an egg is fertilized, the resulting embryo either has an XX or an XY as its 23rd pair – the former develops into a girl, the latter into a boy.

Q Can lifestyle factors affect male fertility?

The simple answer is yes, lifestyle factors can play a big part in male fertility, but the impact of a poor lifestyle will vary from one man to another. For example, some men can drink lots of alcohol and have the worst diet, yet their sperm seem healthy. Others are not so lucky and need to make basic lifestyle changes (see Step 5) to improve the quality and quantity of their sperm.

Research shows that alcohol, cigarettes, cocaine, and marijuana each affect different aspects of the sperm (see pages 78–80). It is important to bear in mind that a couple of nights of heavy drinking, smoking, or taking drugs can affect sperm as much as three months later. If you need to have sperm tests done, a second sample will usually be taken three months after the first, during which time the man has hopefully been in good health – and has been following my recommendations for leading a healthy lifestyle. This will allow doctors to compare the results of the two tests and form an opinion regarding the man's fertility.

You should also be aware that it is not just sperm count and motility that might be affected by unhealthy living. Smoking, drinking, and taking drugs can also damage the genetic material contained in the head of the sperm, which will not be picked up by routine sperm analysis and special tests will need to be done (see page 58).

Q Can illness affect sperm count?

A bout of flu (or any other viral infection) can affect sperm count for several weeks. It takes approximately 100 days for sperm (see opposite page) to become fully mature. So if a man has been unwell, he may be less fertile and if he is having investigations should avoid having a sperm test done until three months after that time, to allow his sperm count to return to what would be a normal level for him.

Q Is it better to have frequent sex or to have sex only on specific days to allow sperm to regenerate?

It appears that conception is more likely to take place if you have frequent sex, rather than abstaining and having sex only on, or just before, the day of ovulation. Aside from the question of whether you have accurately predicted the woman's impending ovulation, a man is likely to have fewer dead or immotile sperm if he has regular intercourse (every two to three days) as his supply is being regularly replenished with new healthy sperm and these are more likely to be able to fertilize an egg.

find out more: **all about sperm**

Once puberty is reached, sperm are manufactured continuously in the two testes at a rate of about 125 million each day. Mature sperm consist of:

■ a head, inside which is a nucleus containing the man's genetic material imprinted on 23 chromosomes. One of these chromosomes is the sex chromosome and will determine the sex of a child (see opposite).

■ a middle section which contains the necessary energy source to make the sperm motile.

■ a long tail to enable it to swim fast and in a straight line.

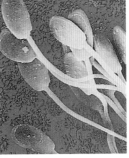

Sperm swim at a rate of 3mm per hour propelled along by their long tails. After ejaculation into the female reproductive tract, only about 1 million make it as far as the cervix, and only about 200 get as far as the fallopian tubes.

sperm **counts**

When semen is analysed (see page 56), the sperm count is considered normal if:

■ there are at least 20 million sperm per ml of seminal fluid

■ there are 15 per cent or more normal-shaped sperm (according to World Health Organization guidelines)

■ the sperm demonstrate normal motility (see page 56)

■ 2–4ml of semen is produced

Acrosome cap *Head* *Midpiece containing mitochondria (energy-providing structures)*

Tail

Up to 1,500 sperm per second are produced in each testicle, and about 250–500 million are expelled every ejaculate.

Q Which medications can affect fertility?

Conditions such as inflammatory bowel disease, urinary tract infection, high blood pressure, and epilepsy may be treated using medication that affects fertility, depending on which drug is used. Ask your GP or specialist for more information. Similarly, you should consult an expert if you require or have recently taken anti-malaria treatment. If you are taking any prescription medication, you should check with your doctor to see if it can affect your fertility, as some drugs can affect sperm production while others may cause problems with sexual performance, including erectile difficulties. On no account should you stop taking medication without seeking a doctor's advice. Luckily, in many cases, alternative drugs that do not effect fertility can be prescribed to treat your condition.

Q Can urological problems have an impact on fertility?

If you have any of the following symptoms, or any other unexplained urological symptoms, consult a doctor:
- pain on urination
- a frequent need to urinate
- getting up regularly during the night to urinate
- blood in the urine
- any unusual or smelly discharge from the penis.

Q Which medical conditions **affect male fertility?**

Some underlying medical conditions can affect a man's fertility. Most commonly, they result in low sperm count (oligozoospermia) but the absence of sperm (azoospermia) can also occur. Certain medical conditions can also lead to erectile dysfunction. See pages 57–59 for more on male subfertility and what can be done to help. The following are just some of the medical conditions that can result in male subfertility.

medical conditions that may have an impact on fertility	
condition	effect on fertility
Epilepsy	Antiepileptic drugs may affect libido and sperm count in some men.
Mumps	If you contracted mumps after puberty or as an adult, you may have developed orchitis, or testicular inflammation, and this may have affected your ability to produce sperm.
Diabetes	This can cause erectile problems.
High blood pressure	Men with high blood pressure find it more difficult to get an erection. In addition, certain drugs called calcium channel blockers which are used to treat this condition may impair the sperm's ability to fertilize the egg.
Surgery, for example to repair an inguinal hernia	This can accidentally block the vas deferens and there can be resulting damage to the blood–testis barrier, which means that blood and testicular tissue come into contact (see page 58). This can then impact on sperm production.
Vasectomy reversal	A vasectomy reversal is not always successful and is not recommended after 5 years. In addition, some men produce antibodies to the sperm following a vasectomy and these attack the sperm even after reversal.

There are several medical conditions you could be suffering from, including a sexually transmitted infection (see pages 18–19), a urinary tract infection, or a more serious condition such as diabetes, and all of these could harm your fertility if they are left untreated. Furthermore, if you have a sexually transmitted infection, you risk damaging your partner's fertility as well.

Q Does being overweight affect male fertility?

Women who are overweight are known to be less fertile than those of normal weight (see page 13), and it is now known that men who are overweight also have an increased risk of being infertile. Research has shown that the more overweight a man is, the more his fertility appears to be impaired. A man who is obese according to the body mass index (BMI of 30 and above) may be only half as fertile as a man with a BMI within the normal range (20–25) – see page 13. He is also more likely to have sperm with fragmented DNA (see page 58), which leads to an increased risk of miscarriage of the fetus.

Doctors are still unsure about why a higher body weight leads to a decrease in fertility, but one theory is that the increased amounts of fat deposited around the genital area of an overweight man could raise his body temperature and as a result reduce the number and motility of healthy sperm being produced.

condition	effect on fertility
Some sexually transmitted infections, such as chlamydia and gonorrhoea	These can cause conditions such as prostatitis, urethritis, and epididymitis. As a result, ducts such as the urethra, vas deferens, or epididymis can become inflamed and subsequently blocked, resulting in irreversible damage to a man's fertility.
Varicocele	This is a condition that is similar to varicose veins and affects the testicular area. It can affect sperm production as a result of reduced blood flow to the affected testicle.
Certain (rare) chromosomal abnormalities	These can cause infertility, either because they result in congenital problems (such as absence of the vas deferens, which is associated with cystic fibrosis) or because there is an absence of sperm (azoospermia). This latter condition may be caused, for example, by Sertoli-cell-only syndrome or by Klinefelter's syndrome (both of which result in the inability to produce sperm).
Retrograde ejaculation	Instead of being propelled through the urethra and out of the penis, the sperm is pushed backwards into the bladder. Surgery can now be used to recover this sperm and, using assisted conception, fertilization of an egg can still take place (see page 155).
Sporting injury	In a contact sport such as rugby or football, a bad accident involving a kick to the groin area can damage the testes' ability to produce sperm.
Torsion or twisting of the testis	If the spermatic cord from which the testis is suspended in the scrotum becomes twisted then the blood supply to the testis can be cut off, causing severe pain. The condition is potentially serious and, if it is not treated immediately, may result in permanent damage to the testis, thereby affecting production of sperm. However, fertility should not be affected as the remaining testis is able to produce sufficient sperm.

Q Can men with erectile problems be helped?

Men with erectile or ejaculatory problems (see pages 72–73) can be helped, assuming their sperm count and sperm quality are acceptable. Depending on the cause of the problem, sperm can be retrieved surgically and ICSI/IVF (see Step 9) used to achieve a pregnancy, or the man can be treated with drugs to stimulate an erection.

In men with retrograde ejaculation (see page 53), drugs can be prescribed that may reverse the problem and lead to normal ejaculation. If that does not work, then sperm can be retrieved and isolated, and intrauterine insemination (IUI) can be attempted (see pages 147–148).

Q How long should we wait before we seek help for fertility problems?

I advise couples who are having problems conceiving to seek help together from the start. It is very frustrating for both when one partner (usually the woman) undergoes investigative tests, only to discover some weeks or months later that, irrespective of whether she has a problem, her partner now needs to undergo tests as well. So, if you have been trying to conceive for a year, or six months if the female partner is over 35, you should both seek specialist help. Ideally, semen tests should be repeated after three months – unless the first test is clearly normal (see page 51) to allow for variations in sperm count and quality.

Q Who can a man go to for help?

Many men I see are unclear about who to consult when it comes to their fertility. While women know to go and see a gynaecologist, men are never sure who to approach, and as the subject of fertility is still taboo among men, they are often lost for advice. If you decide you want to get a sperm test done it is better – if you can – to go to a fertility clinic where the sample will get sent to a laboratory specializing in semen analysis. You will have to pay, but the results you get will be detailed and highly informative.

A test done through your GP will cost you nothing. However, the sample may be sent to the pathology laboratory at a nearby hospital and these results will probably give you a crude sperm count and not much more. Ideally, the test will be done at the local fertility clinic, so try to get a referral earlier, rather than later, and be prepared for NHS waiting lists. If you opt for private treatment, this problem is unlikely to occur, and you will be able to ask where and when the sperm test will be done.

If the semen analysis comes back and there is a problem, you should then see either an appropriately trained gynaecologist in a reproductive medicine clinic (who will be used to dealing with both men and women) or a urologist (if you have urological or erectile/ejaculatory problems), or a clinical andrologist (who specializes in all problems specifically linked to men's reproduction).

Q When should a sample be given?

A sperm sample is usually done following three days of abstinence from sex. Not more, because after this time a sample would have a higher proportion of dead or immotile sperm (which is why conception is more likely to take place if you have frequent sex). And not less, because if you have recently had sex, your sperm sample might not be as full of sperm as it could be, and this would give an artificially low result.

Q Why are sperm counts declining?

It seems that average sperm counts are in decline in the developed world. Although semen analysis is probably more accurate now than it once was, which may account for some of the differences in sperm counts compared to 50 years ago, it does appear that there are a variety of factors (including the increased amount of oestrogenic compounds in our drinking water) that may be affecting sperm production. It is difficult to give a precise figure for average sperm count now compared to 50 years ago, and to provide precise causes – if indeed there is a problem – but there is no doubt that more men are coming forward with fertility problems than before. This is probably due to a cultural shift, and an increased awareness and acceptance that men can be the cause of a couple's fertility problems.

Zita's **tip**

Lifestyle changes are key for helping men to **improve their sperm parameters**.

Q Can **everyday activities** affect sperm counts?

Some of the things that you do as part of your everyday life may present some degree of risk to your fertility.

Mobile phones This is an area that gives cause for concern among my patients. A recent study was published that claimed to have found that men who carried their mobile phones in their trouser pockets and were heavy phone users had lower sperm counts and less motile sperm than men who did not use their phones in this way. However, the study was small and there were too many other possible factors that could have contributed to the findings, so it did not tally with the weight of evidence from other studies that have failed to find any conclusive impact on sperm count or motility as a result of heavy mobile phone use.

Computer laptops I frequently get asked by male patients whether their habit of sitting with a laptop balancing on their lap could be affecting their fertility, as a result of the heat that is emitted from the base of the computer. A recent study whose findings were published in Europe's leading journal of reproductive medicine shows that when a group of healthy men aged 21 to 35 placed the laptops on their lap for one hour, their scrotal temperature increased by nearly one degree. Although the rise was temporary, if it occurs at sufficiently close intervals, recovery time may

not be enough, and irreversible damage to sperm production may occur. So, until more is known about the effects of heat from laptops, it is best that men limit the use of them when they are placed on laps.

Heat In order for sperm production to continue efficiently, it is important that the testes do not become too hot (or too cold, for that matter). Men who work in very hot environments, or who wear very tight clothing for lengthy periods of time, such as the lycra shorts worn by professional cyclists, can find that their sperm production is adversely affected because their scrotum has no way of cooling down. (In cold temperatures, the scrotum contracts and the testes are simply drawn up into the body to keep them at the correct temperature, so sperm production is less affected than it is by constant excessive heat.)

Environmental toxins Sperm production is known to be affected by certain toxins present in the environment. At low doses, these are not harmful but the fertility of men who work or come into regular contact with these toxins could be affected. Toxic metals that can be harmful include lead, cadmium, and mercury, and toxic chemicals include the pesticides dibromochloropropane, chlordecone, and ethylene debromide, and glycol ethers (used in paints, adhesives, and inks).

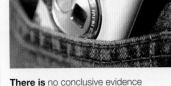

There is no conclusive evidence that mobile phones affect fertility.

Heat generated by laptops on laps can increase scrotal temperature.

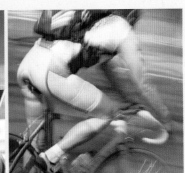

Lycra cycling shorts can also cause the scrotum to overheat.

find out more: **semen analysis**

In the past, semen analysis tested only for numbers of sperm, whereas nowadays it tests for much more, including motility (ability to move and swim quickly) as well as morphology (formation). Poor motility (asthenozoospermia) can mean sperm are unable to swim in a straight line or are unable to swim fast enough. Sperm are graded into any of four levels of motility (this is called progression):

- In level A the sperm show rapid progression in a straight line.
- In level B they have slow progression but with erratic movement.
- In level C they are non-progressive: twitching but not advancing.
- In level D they are immotile and do not move at all.

Sperm will be graded according to what percentage is in each level. Normal levels of motility require at least 25 per cent to be in level A or 50 per cent to be in levels A and B combined. If more than 50 per cent are in levels C and/or D, then the man has a fertility issue.

Sperm counts reveal the actual number of sperm a man is producing. When the count is low (fewer than 20 million per ml) this is referred to as oligozoospermia, whereas azoospermia refers to a complete lack of measurable sperm.

lifestyle impact **on motility**

Poor motility can be a result of lifestyle factors such as:
- drug use
- heavy alcohol use
- smoking
- free radicals in diet.

If you find that your sperm are affected in this way, you should read Steps 5 and 6 to find out what measures you can take to improve your lifestyle and therefore the motility of your sperm.

take a look at sperm morphology

Sperm can be misshapen in many ways. Their heads can vary in size and shape – there can even be two heads – and there can be defects in the middle and tail sections of sperm as well (the tails are sometimes curled round, for example, which prevents them from swimming forwards). High numbers of abnormal-looking sperm (teratozoospermia) will reduce a man's fertility and make conception more difficult.

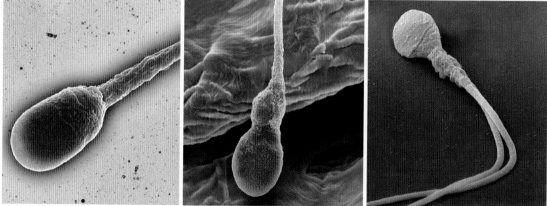

Normal sperm will move with rapid progression in a straight line.

Sperm heads can be misshapen and this will affect their ability to swim.

Motility will be severely impaired if a sperm has two tails.

Q My sperm count has been described as "moderately low". What does this mean?

Moderate oligozoospermia means that you have some functionally normal sperm. In the first instance, both you and your partner should look at ways of improving your general health to give yourselves the best chance of maximizing your fertility.

Subsequently, intrauterine insemination (IUI) may be considered using preparations of 3 to 5 million progressively motile sperm (see page 56). Your partner will need to have at least one of her fallopian tubes fully functioning and will need to be undergoing ovarian stimulation (see pages 146–147). In such conditions, three to four cycles of IUI result in conception in 15 to 30 per cent of couples.

If 1 to 2 million motile sperm are present in a prepared sample of semen, IVF would be the next option (see pages 147–159).

Q I have a very low sperm count – is there any hope for conception?

When a sperm count shows there are fewer than 5 million sperm per ml this is referred to as severe oligozoospermia. The cause is often genetic. Around 7 to 10 per cent of men with oligozoospermia are shown to have a genetic defect – such as a deletion of certain genetic material on their Y chromosome – when tested. This may make it more likely that their infertility could be passed on to male children and may also increase the risk of certain birth defects.

Intracytoplasmic sperm injection, known as ICSI (see page 155), combined with IVF, would be used if low numbers of motile sperm were detected (indeed, only one viable sperm is actually needed for this method to succeed). The ability to isolate a single sperm and inject it into the egg, first performed in Belgium in about 1992, has been a major advance in treating male infertility.

Q What is azoospermia?

Azoospermia is the term used to describe the condition where there is an absence of sperm in seminal fluid. Azoospermia can be either non-obstructive or obstructive. Non-obstructive is caused most commonly either by an

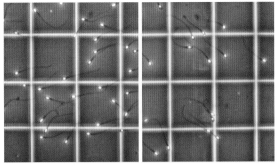

Normal sperm count   Low sperm count

undescended testicle or testes (cryptorchidism), by a hormonal or genetic abnormality such as Klinefelter's syndrome, or by damage following chemotherapy or radiotherapy. Men with this form of azoospermia should have genetic testing, because around 15 to 30 per cent will have sex chromosome aneuploidy or chromosomal anomalies (see page 58).

In obstructive azoospermia, sperm production and testicular size are normal but there is testicular obstruction caused, for example, by a failed vasectomy reversal or by a chlamydia or gonorrhoea infection (see page 18). When this occurs, spermatozoa (some of which may be immature) can be retrieved surgically under local anaesthetic. In one technique called PESA (percutaneous epididymal sperm aspiration), sperm is taken directly from the coiled tube in the testis called the epididymis. Alternatively, using TESE (testicular sperm extraction) sperm is taken from a small portion of tissue from the testes. Sperm is then injected directly into the egg using ICSI. The results with these procedures are similar to – or sometimes even better than – cycles where ejaculated sperm is used. Fortunately, vasectomy reversal will restore sperm in semen in 80 to 90 per cent of men, and pregnancies occur in 40 to 50 per cent of couples after one to two years.

Although azoospermia is uncommon, 75 per cent of men with this condition now have the possibility of biological fatherhood thanks to improved assisted conception techniques, and ICSI in particular.

Q What else can sperm tests check for?

Sperm tests have become increasingly sophisticated and can now be used to test for a whole range of factors that can potentially affect fertility. These tests would not necessarily be part of a standard NHS test and need to be paid for, but they can reveal invaluable information. This might include:

▪ Acidity of semen (sperm is usually alkaline with a pH between 7.2 and 8).

▪ Agglutination: this means that motile sperm stick to one another and usually indicates the presence of anti-sperm antibodies (proteins that coat sperm and bind to cervical mucus, preventing sperm from moving towards an egg or fertilizing it). If sperm are sticking to each other, a MAR (mixed agglutination reaction) test will be needed. In healthy sperm this should show less than 50 per cent binding and should not affect fertility.

▪ Presence of antibodies: these are not usually present in semen, however they may be caused by injury or surgery such as vasectomy reversal or hernia repair, where a breakdown in the blood–testis barrier allows blood and testicular tissue to mix. When antibodies are present at relatively high levels, fertility may be affected. As well as preventing sperm from moving, they may coat the sperm heads, making it difficult for them to recognize an egg and fertilize it.

▪ Concentration of round cells (these are either immature sperm cells or white blood cells). A raised concentration of these may indicate an infection, which if serious can result in permanent damage.

Q What does more advanced sperm analysis involve?

Further sperm tests are now available that are highly detailed. These are still controversial and as a result are not offered routinely, if at all, even in the majority of fertility clinics. You should check if your clinic offers tests for the following:

▪ DNA fragmentation. This test is common in the USA but rarely available here. DNA is the genetic material carried on our chromosomes, and although the egg can still be fertilized by sperm that has some low-level

Zita's **tip**

Don't give up hope if you get poor sperm test results – there will be **lots that can be done** to help.

DNA damage, more serious damage means that either the sperm cannot fertilize the egg, or the resulting embryo is incompatible with life, and the pregnancy miscarries. Scientists can now screen sperm for DNA fragmentation or chromosomal abnormalities. Between 2 and 13 per cent of sperm are expected to be genetically abnormal, and although age can increase the figure, environmental and lifestyle factors, including cigarette smoking and alcohol, can also significantly affect the percentage of abnormal sperm. When DNA damage is not genetic in origin, it may be caused by free radicals in our diet and environment (see page 55). But with a change in lifestyle, men can often reduce the amount of abnormal sperm and improve their fertility.

▪ Aneuploidy. This occurs when there is one or more extra or missing chromosomes. This leads to genetic abnormalities, some of which are incompatible with life; others, such as trisomy 21 (or Down's syndrome) will result in a fetal abnormality. There is an increased aneuploidy rate in sperm with fragmented DNA and there are two highly specialized tests that can determine this: a sperm chromatin dispersion (SCD) test and a fluorescence in situ hybridization (FISH) test.

▪ P34H levels. Research has shown that the protein P34H plays a key role in fertilization and that low or nonexistent levels of the protein on the surface of sperm occur in a significant number of subfertile men. The protein is needed to enable fertilization to take place, so its low/absent levels could throw light on certain cases of previously unexplained infertility. This is a new test and, although it is available in the US, it is currently available only in a few clinics in the UK.

Q Are there any male fertility tests that might be needed other than semen analysis?

Yes, in fact semen analysis really is only part of the story. Further tests might include hormone analysis, which involves a simple blood test to check for levels of the key sex hormones: FSH, LH, testosterone, and prolactin. Results falling either side of the expected range indicate hormonal imbalance which can be treated with hormone-replacement drugs. If levels of FSH and LH are high and levels of testosterone are low, you may have testicular failure. In this case examination of a sample of tissue from the testes will help determine whether or not

case**study**

No problems were found when Stuart's partner Jane had fertility tests – then it was his turn. Stuart freely admits he found the tests quite an ordeal.

Stuart I was dreading the day I would have to do the test. You hear accounts of other men going but never imagine you might have to. On the morning I went to the clinic I kept thinking what if I can't produce a sample or what if I bump into somebody I know? When I arrived the nurses were great but I felt incredibly self-conscious, knowing that everybody knew what I was about to do. I went off to a little room and managed to perform but I felt really tense, which doesn't help. It felt surreal as I listened to other people's conversations outside the door. I wanted to hide my specimen when I came out and was very conscious of the full waiting room. As I left, I kept thinking what if there is no sperm? What if I can't have children? What next? How will Jane take it?

After five days I went back for my results, which looked so complicated. I wanted the answer to be simple: can I have kids or not? My GP explained the results to me. My sperm count was good: 70 million. But motility was poor and the number with abnormal shapes was very high. I was told that IUI was the route we should go down, but that it would take time to conceive with these results.

We have decided not to rush. To start, my lifestyle needs to change: I smoke and drink and am under a lot of stress so I will address these issues then get another test done in four months' time. If the results don't improve then we will consider our options.

It is easy to tell a man to go and get a sperm test done, but men dread doing this and need a lot of support from their partners and medical staff.

it is possible to retrieve sperm (see page 57) for use in intracytoplasmic sperm injection (ICSI – see page 155).

Beyond this, further tests may be recommended to establish whether or not there is damage to the testes, or any other physiological damage, or genetic defects. Cell culture can identify infection, which may result in reduced testosterone production and diminished sperm count. Ultrasound scanning can be used to check the physiological health of the scrotum, testes, epididymis, prostate, and seminal vesicles. Finally, blood tests may be done in order to obtain a genetic evaluation, as about 4 per cent of men with a sperm count lower than 5 million per ml and up to 15 per cent of those with no sperm have a chromosomal abnormality.

Q What are the psychological effects of male infertility?

Men associate their fertility so much with their virility – and our culture encourages this – that it is always a big shock and a huge psychological blow when a man discovers that there is something wrong. He often feels he has let his partner down and feels immensely guilty that he is putting her through an ordeal that he perceives as being "his fault". Consequently, it is normal for him to feel depressed and diminished as a person. These feelings will be accentuated if the quality of his sperm cannot be improved and if he and his partner need fertility treatment to conceive. Problems of impotence and/or anger at the apparent unfairness of the situation are also common and in such circumstances the couple's relationship often comes under strain.

Support from the female partner is essential in this situation, as is seeking expert medical advice, in order to help the man to stay positive. It is important that a couple keeps talking to each other, although the man may find it difficult under the circumstances. Seeing a counsellor or therapist can also be useful.

Men should be encouraged by the fact that a diagnosis of infertility, thanks to medical advances, need not be as devastating as it would have been in the past. Indeed, much can be done to enable men to father children naturally or with assisted conception (see Step 9). So if you find yourself in the increasingly common situation of having a fertility problem, you should bear in mind that there is still every chance that you will be able to father a child.

questionnaire: **what do you know about male fertility?**

Having read this section, you should now be able to make an **informed review of your potential** for fathering a child and identify the things you can do to **positively influence your chances**. Score 1 for each "yes" and gain some insight into your fertility level

Have you ever had a sexually transmitted infection?

yes ☐   **no** ☐

Untreated STIs can lead to blocked ducts and infertility, and can also affect female fertility as well (see pages 18–19).

Do you have any erectile or ejaculatory problems?

yes ☐   **no** ☐

These are reasonably common. See pages 72–73 for possible causes and treatment options.

Are you over 45?

yes ☐   **no** ☐

Sperm quality deteriorates with age and by 45 you will have a higher proportion of abnormal sperm (see page 48).

Do you suffer from medical conditions such as epilepsy, diabetes, or high blood pressure?

yes ☐   **no** ☐

Some underlying medical conditions can affect male fertility. Men who suffer from epilepsy often have fertility problems, and treatment for diabetes and high blood pressure can cause erectile problems and so impact on fertility (see page 52). Discuss these conditions with your specialist. Score 1 point for each.

Do you take regular medication?

yes ☐   **no** ☐

Certain medication affects fertility or erectile function (see page 52). Check with your doctor.

Did you have mumps in puberty or adulthood?

yes ☐   **no** ☐

This may have affected your ability to produce sperm.

Have you ever had a severe injury to the groin/testicles?

yes ☐   **no** ☐

Sperm production may have been harmed (see page 53).

Have you had an operation for undescended testis or testes?

yes ☐   **no** ☐

This may have led to impaired sperm production. You may want to consider having a sperm test to check.

Have you had a vasectomy reversal or surgery for an inguinal hernia?

yes ☐   **no** ☐

Both procedures carry the risk of damage to the blood–testis barrier (see page 52).

Do you work in a very hot environment or one where you are in regular contact with toxic materials?

yes ☐ **no** ☐

Both factors are known to affect production of sperm (see page 55).

Have you been trying for a baby and having lots of unprotected sex for over a year?

yes ☐ **no** ☐

Even if you are already a father, problems may have arisen since your child was born.

Are you having timed sex (mainly at/around ovulation) and abstaining at other times of the month?

yes ☐ **no** ☐

Research indicates that this decreases your chances of conceiving (see page 51).

your**score**

0–3 Even with such a low score, you should ask yourself whether any of your "yes" answers are the result of something that could affect your fertility. Don't assume all is fine, particularly if you have been trying to conceive for at least a year.

4–7 Your fertility may be compromised. You should investigate whether some of the areas of concern are affecting your chances of biologically fathering a child. It may be time for you to get a sperm test done and to consider whether your diet and lifestyle could also be improved in order to maximize your fertility.

8–12 You may well have a fertility problem and should consult a specialist to investigate further. Much can be done to help men who are diagnosed as infertile to father a child, but the sooner you seek help, the better your chances of success.

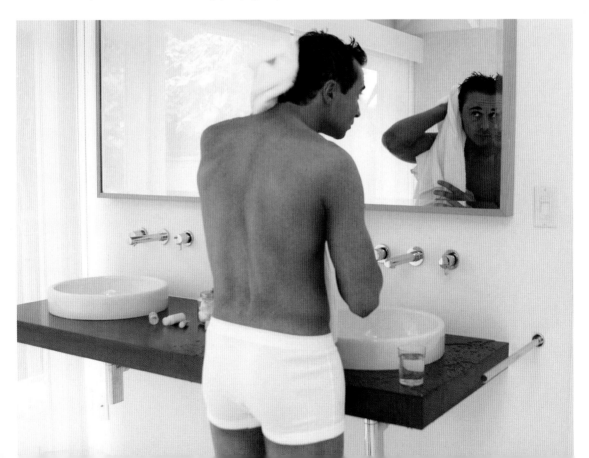

"Don't let the fact that you are trying for a baby spoil the **fun of having sex** – the key is communication: **keep talking** to each other"

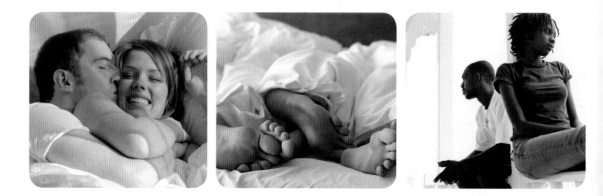

step**four**
sex and passion

Your questions answered on:

step four: **sex and passion**

" Many couples lose the **spontaneity and passion** in their sex life when they are trying for a baby. Yet it is vital for the long-term health of any relationship to regain this **fun and intimacy**. This step addresses some of the questions about sex that have an impact, not only on a couple's happiness but also on their **chance of conceiving** "

Q How often should we be having sex?

Couples who are trying to conceive often fall into the habit of having sex only around the time when they think the woman is fertile. Before long, this becomes an unspoken pattern between them. For a few days every month, they feel it is "worth" having sex, even though they may have intercourse only a couple of times in that phase. The rest of the month, nothing happens at all because there's "no point". Yet, this is harmful on two counts. First, if you are trying to conceive you need to maximize your chances by having a lot of sex. Secondly, if you are having sex only during a short period of time each month, by the time you have sex again the following month, the sperm waiting to be released are old. As a result, a higher proportion will either be less motile, abnormal (see page 51), or dead. It is better for a man's fertility if sperm are regularly renewed through ejaculation. If ejaculation does not happen very often, the chances of conception will be affected.

Given that the egg can only be fertilized in the first 24 hours after ovulation, and sperm can survive for an average of two to three days (potentially longer) in the female reproductive tract, it is important that regular quantities of fresh, active, healthy sperm are present and ready to attempt fertilization. So, ideally, you should be having sex every two or three days throughout your cycle, not just around the time when you think you are fertile.

Q Does sexual desire change when couples try to conceive?

Around 90 per cent of the couples I see agree that their sex lives are affected one way or another by trying to get pregnant. In the early days, many find that their sex

life is enhanced because it can be liberating not to have to use any form of contraception. Indeed, it is quite likely that this will never have been the case before. Most women spend their entire reproductive lives trying not to get pregnant, so suddenly not having to worry about this can feel very erotic and sexually liberating.

For other couples, however, and these are the majority of those I see, their sex life starts to suffer soon after they decide to try for a baby. Typically, this happens after four or five months, when pregnancy has not occurred and anxiety and tension start to creep in, but the deterioration can begin at any time if sex becomes "planned" from the start. So, if you are in this situation, and your sex life and libido are not what they were, you are far from being alone. Let me reassure you, with a little extra effort and communication between you both, you can get your sex life back on track.

Q I'm worried that sex has become "baby" sex, rather than fun sex. What should we do?

Sex is a habit: the more you have it, the more you are used to having it, and the more you are likely to want it. If you are now in the situation where the only reason to have sex is because it might lead to a pregnancy, then the chances are you have got out of the habit of having it simply when you feel like it. As well as impacting on your chances of conceiving, this sort of "baby" sex starts to have an effect on your relationship. Not only does sex become artificial and done to order, but your general physical relationship with your partner also starts to feel contrived and self-conscious because you are no longer used to giving and receiving pleasure, and to sharing intimacy regularly and spontaneously. In my experience, if you lose

Q Which hormones play a role in **sexual desire**?

Many individual hormones interact to affect how much sexual desire we experience, although how this works is not yet fully understood. The hormones oestrogen and testosterone play a key part but other hormones are also important to our sexual well-being.

Oestrogen This is produced in the ovaries and is important for vaginal lubrication and sexual pleasure. Oestrogen levels are significantly higher in women of reproductive age. This is one reason why post-menopausal women experience decreased vaginal lubrication and reduced libido. Some women report that their maximum sexual desire coincides with the most fertile time of the cycle when there is an abundance of oestrogenic secretions, which is favourable to sperm survival.

Testosterone This hormone, produced in the testes in men and in the ovaries in women, is responsible for sex drive in both men and women. Men's levels of testosterone start to drop as they get older, leading to a drop in their desire for sex. Similarly, women's levels of testosterone are highest before the age of 20 and drop thereafter.

Serotonin The gut secretes over 95 per cent of the body's serotonin. This chemical plays a vital role in the regulation of mood, including anger, and also regulates sleep, temperature, and sexuality. Women need serotonin in order to experience feelings of comfort, sexual satisfaction, and relaxation.

Dopamine This is a chemical released by the hypothalamus. Its main function is to inhibit the release of the hormone prolactin from the pituitary gland. Dopamine is commonly associated with the pleasure system of the brain because it provides feelings of enjoyment from experiences such as eating or having sex.

Oxytocin This hormone is made in the hypothalamus and is secreted from the pituitary gland. It is involved in social recognition and bonding. It also has an anti-stress function in that it reduces blood pressure and

levels of the stress hormone cortisol, therefore reducing anxiety and increasing tolerance of pain (see page 84).

Both men and women release oxytocin during orgasm. In women, oxytocin is secreted as a result of massage and touch, stimulation of the nipples, and contractions of the uterus during orgasm. Oxytocin effects are linked to the production of oestrogen: as oestrogen levels rise, the effects of oxytocin also increase. It's no surprise that women are often extremely sensitive to touch and can be aroused much more quickly when they at their most fertile and their oestrogen levels are at their highest, compared to other times of the month when they are less fertile and have lower oestrogen and oxytocin levels.

Women and men who are not touched much by their partners have lower levels of oxytocin and this can result in higher levels of cortisol in the body. It can also lead to a gradual deterioration of their relationship because the bonding role that oxytocin plays is gradually reduced.

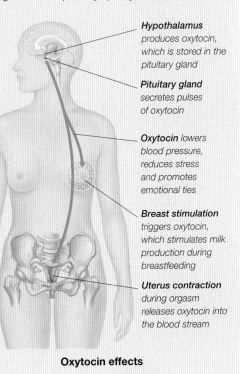

Hypothalamus produces oxytocin, which is stored in the pituitary gland

Pituitary gland secretes pulses of oxytocin

Oxytocin lowers blood pressure, reduces stress and promotes emotional ties

Breast stimulation triggers oxytocin, which stimulates milk production during breastfeeding

Uterus contraction during orgasm releases oxytocin into the blood stream

Oxytocin effects

this emotional connection with your partner, this eventually leads to you being less open and communicative with each other. The result is that your relationship ends up suffering. Talking to each other about your feelings is often the key to resolving these issues (see page 68).

Q How much does my partner need to know about my monthly cycle?

One of the things I always say to women is that there is no need to tell their man absolutely everything about their menstrual cycle. If possible, for example, I advise them to avoid informing their partners on details such as what their secretions are doing or what their temperature is that day, because on the whole it is not conducive to sexual arousal. Indeed, many men have told me that it is a complete turn-off. The fact is, he doesn't need to know as much as you do, particularly if you are trying to get him in the mood for sex.

Clearly, if you are going through fertility treatment together, you will both end up knowing more than you ever thought you would on all aspects of male and female reproduction. And I realize that it's important for men to be well informed so that they can really support their partners as they go through this together, but there are many opportunities for women to discuss the subject without necessarily going into minute detail and without doing so at inappropriate times.

Q What are the main triggers for sex in men and women?

You each need to ask yourselves what normally triggers your desire for sex. Ignoring the fact that you are trying for a baby, try to gain awareness of what makes you want to have sex. The answers will doubtless be very different depending on whether you are a man or a woman. Spontaneous desire for sex is common among men. In addition, while most men respond to visual

stimuli and to specific moods and feelings, others need to think about or even enact certain fantasies to become aroused. Women, on the other hand, respond to mood, verbal communication with their partner, a feeling of intimacy and trust and of being loved and wanted. Visual stimuli are less important, but fantasies can also play a part in women's arousal. Women often do not feel like sex unless they feel relaxed and stress-free, whereas men often use sex as a form of stress relief.

The reality is that, for many women, the trigger for sex is not watching a steamy DVD. Instead, it is more likely to involve her man cooking a meal and doing the washing-up without needing to be asked, or bringing her breakfast in bed in the morning.

Sometimes "triggers" for sex do not need to be explained – indeed, if they involve fantasies, it may be better not to. But it can also help to discuss the triggers with your partner, particularly if you are in a relationship where your sex life has deteriorated to the point where you are going through the motions for the sake of making a baby (see page 69).

Q Is a man always able to have sex if his partner is willing?

This is one of the big myths surrounding sex and it is never more apparent than when a woman decides she needs to have sex because it is her fertile time. Sometimes she is so desperate that she does not expect (or even want) any preamble or mood-setting to get herself and her man aroused. And in any event, she believes that most men are only too eager to have sex if given half a chance, so why bother with the preliminaries? All she is thinking about is the possibility of getting pregnant and any notions of romance have gone out the window.

Yet, for a surprising number of men, being told to perform there and then, as if they are a walking sperm machine, is a complete turn-off and can easily lead to a man being unable to get an erection. Several men have revealed to me that their female partners had sent them texts or emails at work telling them to come home urgently (even making them cancel any plans they might have had) because they have noticed signs of ovulation. Not surprisingly, this resulted in anger and resentment on the part of the man, frustration on the part of the woman, an argument and no sex, sometimes because the man was simply unable to "perform" to order.

Q Are there any reasons why women may be unable to have sex?

Many women who become focused on getting pregnant complain that they feel dry and sex becomes uncomfortable. Unfortunately, all vaginal lubricants, whether water or oil-based (and even saliva), have been shown in rigorous trials to adversely affect sperm. Ideally, avoid using lubricants and aim to spend more time caressing and using foreplay to stimulate your body's own natural lubricating fluids. If this approach does not work, then it is better to use a minimal amount of lubricant on the vaginal lips than to risk getting sore from dry sex.

It is not uncommon for couples to experience sexual difficulties after a few months of trying to conceive when they have previously had a really good sex life. As always, the main thing here is to try to relax and to talk about it with your partner. If you are concerned about dryness, talk to your doctor. It may be related to your age or to hormonal changes. Try to minimize your use of tampons (see page 34) and avoid thongs as these can also be drying. Lifestyle and nutrition changes may be helpful (see Steps 5 and 6).

find out more: **sexual response**

Sexual response can be divided into four phases: the excitement or arousal phase, the plateau phase, orgasm, and the resolution phase, when the body returns to normal. These phases occur in both men and women but with subtle differences. In men, sexual excitement builds rapidly to reach a plateau; in women it is more gradual. In both, arousal peaks at orgasm, which may or may not occur simultaneously.

A woman may have a short plateau phase, followed by a single orgasm; a longer plateau phase and multiple orgasms; or a plateau phase with no orgasm and a much slower resolution phase. Although men may find it hard to relate to this, all of these experiences can be deeply satisfying for a woman. Certainly, women do not need to reach orgasm to have fulfilling sexual intercourse.

The refractory period refers to the time taken before a man is able to become sexually aroused again. Usually, the older a man is, the longer this period will be. Women, on the other hand, do not have a refractory period and, if they are stimulated appropriately, they can go on to have sex and further orgasms very soon after.

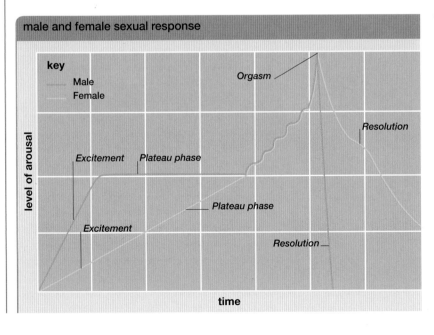

male and female sexual response

key
Male
Female

Orgasm

Resolution

level of arousal

Excitement   Plateau phase

Plateau phase

Excitement

Resolution

time

facts about
orgasm

- The pattern of sexual response varies from one individual to another and from one experience to another.
- Orgasm doubles the heart rate, raises blood pressure, and causes the release of oxytocin.
- Women don't have to reach orgasm to conceive, but men do to ejaculate.

find out more: **restoring harmony**

Relationships often suffer when couples start trying for a baby, particularly if **pregnancy has not happened** after a few months.

I see countless couples whose relationships are under strain and whose sex lives, consequently, are also going through problems. They come to me because they are trying to understand why this is and what they can do about it. Sex and relationships are intricately bound up and, if one area starts to encounter difficulties, the other will as well.

There is a lot of psychobabble talked about sex. People are often led to believe that their childhood is the cause of any sexual problems they might have. While this may be true for some people – and clearly, earlier relationships based on abuse, whether verbal, physical, emotional, or sexual, are extremely harmful – for most people, their sexual problems are recent and temporary, and are due to the fact that their concern about not getting pregnant is causing problems within the relationship.

What are the effects of "baby" sex?

56%

of women in a survey of 500 attending my clinic felt their sex life had been affected by trying to conceive. A few felt this was affected positively (more sex), but the vast majority felt their sex life had been negatively affected.

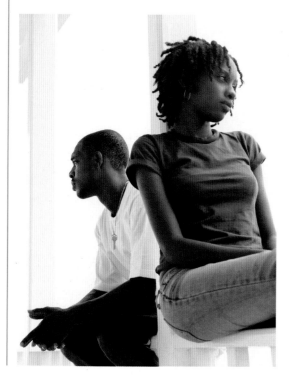

communication problems

We often use sex subconsciously to communicate with our partners: it is a way of expressing feelings, including negative ones. You may avoid sex out of unspoken anger, resentment, or frustration. Yet, by doing so, you are missing out on possible opportunities for getting pregnant. You may also be letting certain issues fester away when they need to be discussed for the long-term health of the relationship.

Ask yourself these questions to see whether your relationship is beginning to suffer:
■ Do you repeatedly have arguments that go nowhere, then go away for a while, only to rear their ugly heads again?
■ Does everything your partner says seem highly personal?
■ Do you overreact to comments from your partner?
■ Do you feel resentful and bitter towards him/her?
It is important to be aware of where you think your relationship is at, because if you think it is suffering, then now is the time to do something about it.

If your sex life and your relationship are being dominated by your plans to become pregnant, now is the time to acknowledge this.

what causes a lack of desire?

Ironically, the time when you should be having sex the most – when you are trying for a baby – is often the time when one or both partners begin to experience a lack of libido and your sex life starts to be affected. Indeed, many couples use the "I'm too tired for sex" excuse, when in fact they are frightened of failure or feeling depressed. Human sexuality is very complex and, in order to feel aroused, you need certain key factors to be in place. You might love and trust your partner, but you may feel a host of other negative emotions that counteract these feelings and lead to you feeling less desire than before.

Negative emotions might include:

■ **Anxiety** If you are a man, you might worry that you are not able to perform on demand, or you might not be as keen as your partner to have a baby but have not been able to tell her. If you are a woman, you might be anxious about why you are still not pregnant and whether you are even able to conceive.

■ **Grief** You might have had a miscarriage in the past or you might be mourning the fact that you may not be able to conceive without fertility treatment.

■ **Stress** You might be feeling under pressure to have sex and to get pregnant (see Steps 5 and 7 for more on stress and the mind–body link).

These and other emotions can easily get in the way of any desire to have sex – or at least the sort of sex you used to enjoy with your partner, when you simply had it because you felt like it. In addition, these emotional issues can contribute to physical problems (see pages 72–73), which in turn result in a reduced desire for sex.

steps to **recovery**

■ Identify why you think your libido has gone down since you started trying for a baby.
■ Discuss your conclusions openly and honestly with your partner.
■ Make time to be together. Share your hopes as well as your fears and disappointments with each other.

case**study**

Richard and Julia had been trying to get pregnant for one year. As the pressure built up, other aspects of their relationship began to fall apart.

Richard It took me a bit longer than Julia to decide that I was ready to have a baby. Although I am 34, I still enjoyed nights out with my friends and was worried about how a baby would impact on our lives.

Within a few months of deciding to start trying the fun and intimacy in our sex life vanished. I started to dread ovulation time as Julia kept a constant dialogue going, describing every intimate detail of what was happening in her body, which quite frankly was a real turn-off. Sex was dictated by Julia depending on her ovulation time and I found it harder and harder to perform to order. When she started getting annoyed about me going out with friends and enjoying a few drinks I began to feel resentful at her expectation that I should give up my social life. I also came to dread going home around the time her period was due. She would dissolve into tears and

depression each month when it started. I didn't dare to tell her when someone at work announced that their partner was pregnant!

Julia felt that I didn't understand and that I didn't want a baby as much as her. It reached the point where the need to conceive was starting to take over the whole of our relationship. At this time we decided we needed help and went to see Zita for some advice on how to rescue our relationship as well as on fertility issues."

After coming to see me, Richard and Julia began to recognize that they need to be more communicative in order to avoid building up unspoken resentment and anger.

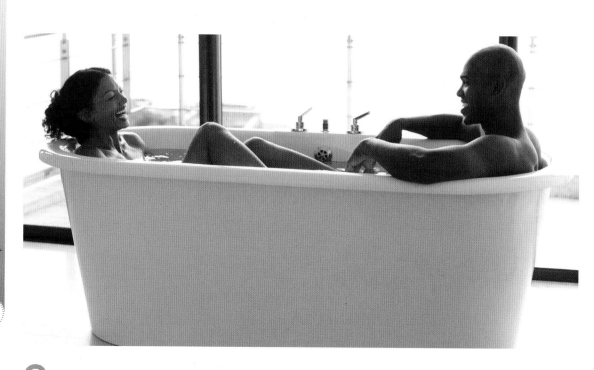

Q How can we revitalize our sex life?

Try to let go of your conscious mind: that it is "the right time" and you must have sex today to get pregnant. Stop worrying about things such as whether you are having sex in the right position or whether too much sperm has just leaked out. Just enjoy the sensation of having sex.

■ Have sex when it feels best for you. If you are exhausted last thing at night, either go to bed earlier or have sex at other times of day.

■ Try to recreate situations that used to get you in the mood for sex. These might include surprise candle-lit dinners at home or having a long, relaxing bath together.

■ Everyday routine can be a passion-killer, so aim to bring in an element of change. A weekend break or even an overnight stay in a nearby hotel can revive your relationship and enable you to rediscover what you were like as a couple before you started trying for a baby.

Zita's **tip**

Be sensitive to **each other's feelings** when you have **conversations about sex**.

Think about creating situations that get you in the mood for sex: when was the last time you had a bath together, for example?

■ Notice and comment on the things you do for each other and enjoy about each other, rather than dwell on disappointments and negative aspects.

Q Does fertility treatment affect a couple's sex life?

It is very common for a couple's sex life to collapse when they realize they need fertility treatment. They have come to equate having sex with making babies and now that this link is no longer there, making love seems pointless. In addition, if one half of the couple has a fertility problem (as opposed to both partners), that person inevitably suffers a major psychological blow. However supportive their partner is, they always feel their masculinity or femininity is deeply affected and this naturally harms their libido.

Yet, it is vital for two important reasons that you do not fall into the trap of no longer bothering to make love. First, you never know: there is so much anecdotal evidence of couples conceiving naturally despite being told that they need fertility treatment to have a child.

I have regularly treated patients over the years who were about to undergo IVF or where the male partner supposedly had a low sperm count, and who spontaneously became pregnant. Secondly, sex is not just about babies. It's about rapport, communication, and pleasure. And it's about your relationship. So even if you need assisted conception in order to get pregnant, remember that sex is an essential part of how you function as an individual and as a couple, and it needs to be maintained for the long-term health and survival of your relationship.

Q Is it normal to feel resentful of a partner's fertility problem?

This can certainly happen, but it is a pointless, destructive feeling and one that can be overcome by becoming aware of certain truths. First, do not race ahead of yourself. Your partner may have a fertility problem, but this does not mean that you will not become parents. Many fertility problems can be overcome and some even resolve themselves without the need for medical intervention. Sometimes, time and patience is all that is required, or a change of diet and lifestyle. I know that is of little comfort to you if all you want is to conceive as soon as possible, but I have come across so many couples who were despondent about their chances of becoming pregnant, yet when they made a few changes to their lives, they conceived a baby.

Secondly, it is vital that you do not lose sight of who your partner is. This is the person you fell in love with. You did not choose your partner because of his or her fertility, but because of a host of qualities you loved and admired and were attracted to. What good is the most fertile person in the world if he or she does not have what it takes to make you happy in the way your partner has up until now? And the last thing your partner needs right now is to feel a failure. He or she needs your complete support and understanding, and to be certain that you will continue to go through life together, whatever happens, as a team.

If you let your disappointment in the situation show, you could not only be harming your chances of conception (through excessive anxiety and pressure) but you could be doing permanent damage to your relationship. Concentrate on what makes you happy as a couple, and on loving each other as you have done in the past, and you will be ready to take on whatever life throws at you.

Q Which **medical problems** affect libido?

Women Some medical and hormonal conditions adversely affect a woman's libido. These include diabetes, cardiovascular or blood pressure problems, hypothyroidism, depression, and anxiety. Pelvic surgery and urological or bowel conditions also make a woman less likely to want sex.

Some medication can reduce a woman's sexual drive and lead to sexual dysfunction if her reduced libido has become a problem for both the woman and her partner. The drugs concerned include certain antidepressants, sedatives, antihistamines, and contraceptive drugs.

Men Various medical conditions, such as heart disease and diabetes, can cause erectile problems (see page 72), and thyroid disease is known to affect some men's sex drive.

Certain medications can have an effect on male libido and sexual function. Antidepressants are the medicines most frequently implicated in causing sexual dysfunction, and this is because they alter the levels of chemicals in the brain. Antihypertensives such as beta blockers are also known to cause problems; around 25 per cent of erectile failure is believed to be caused by these drugs. Other medicines that can have adverse effects on male sexual function include anti-anxiety and insomnia treatment (decreased sex drive); peptic ulcer treatment (decreased sex drive, impotence); and cholesterol-lowering medicines (impotence).

Resolving problems In many instances, treatment of the medical condition helps to resolve libido problems, so it is important to see your doctor for a diagnosis if you have unexplained symptoms. If you suspect that a prescription (or over-the-counter) medication is affecting sexual desire, check the side-effects listed in the pack and if you are at all worried, talk to your doctor. He or she may be able to suggest an alternative. Never stop taking prescription medication without talking to your doctor first.

find out more: **sexual problems**

Both men and women can **experience problems with sex**. These can be caused by a variety of factors, **some physical, some psychological.**

Experiencing sexual problems is something few people are prepared to admit to, yet the reality is that many of us do encounter some issue or other with sex at some point in our lives. Whether it be difficulty getting an erection or reaching orgasm, or that you and your partner experience different levels of desire, it is important to address the issues you encounter together to maximize your chances of conception.

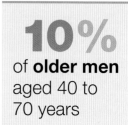

10% of **older men** aged 40 to 70 years

suffer complete erectile dysfunction, yet very few seek medical help.

men's sexual problems

The most common male sexual difficulty, and one that affects fertility, is erectile dysfunction (ED). This is the repeated inability to get or keep an erection firm enough for sexual intercourse to take place.

Erectile dysfunction is either physical or psychological in origin. In the former, it is more often found in older men because they are more likely to be suffering from conditions such as diabetes, high blood pressure, and clogged arteries, which are known to affect sexual function. Reduced libido can also be caused by certain medications or medical conditions, such as heart problems and diabetes (see page 71).

Experts estimate that psychological factors such as stress, guilt, depression, low self-esteem, and fear of sexual failure account for 10 to 20 per cent of ED cases. Other possible causes are smoking and drinking, which restrict blood flow to veins and arteries and damage egg and sperm production.

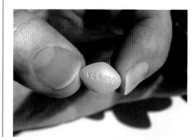

Sildenafil *(Viagra)* is a well-known drug therapy that helps many men to achieve and maintain an erection.

Treatment If you suffer from this form of sexual difficulty, treatment will depend on the cause of the problem and how long you have suffered from it. If it is a recent occurrence, the chances are that, unless you have recently developed a medical condition (see pages 52–53), your ED is more likely to be psychological in nature. Consulting a urologist (your GP can refer you) will help you discover whether there is any underlying systemic or medical issue. If nothing is discovered, you should look at possible psychological and lifestyle causes and decide if you need to make any changes.

■ Assess whether you are under excessive stress: identify which areas of your life are causing this and find ways of improving the situation (see Step 5).

■ Make lifestyle changes: stopping smoking, exercising more, losing weight, and reducing alcohol intake may be enough to solve the problem.

■ You may need drug therapy, if only temporarily. Sildenafil citrate (Viagra) relaxes blood vessels in the penis to increase blood flow and produce an erection.

■ Vacuum devices and surgery are more invasive treatment options that would only be considered if all the above had failed. However, they can successfully treat ED in severe cases or where there is a physical cause of the problem.

You should be reassured that, although erectile dysfunction and other problems of impotence are more common as men get older, they are by no means an inevitable part of ageing.

women's sexual problems

Women may suffer from a range of sexual problems or sexual difficulties. The most common of these is poor libido, followed by difficulty in getting or staying aroused, difficulty or inability to achieve orgasm, and pain during intercourse. Sexual response for a woman depends on a complex interaction of factors, including her health, physiology, emotions, experiences, beliefs, lifestyle, and relationships. If one area is affected, sexual drive, arousal, and satisfaction can suffer. Emotional difficulties can encompass anxiety, stress, or depression and these often lead to sexual problems. Similarly, if a woman has negative feelings about her body, these can also cause difficulties. Unless there is a specific health factor at the root of the problem, a woman usually needs to address the psychological and relationship issues in order to improve her sex life.

Treatment If you are troubled by any form of sexual problem, first of all you need to make sure you are not suffering from any underlying condition or are not taking any medication that could affect your libido or your ability to get aroused and lubricated (see pages 20–25). Next, you need to address relationship issues that could be causing a problem (see below). Finally, assess whether any part of your lifestyle (such as lack of sleep or excessive stress – see Step 5) could be damaging your sex life.

Venus and Mars

- Women need: more stimulation, slow foreplay, cuddling and kissing, romance, emotional sharing.
- Men need: spontaneity, physical passion, playful sex, visual stimulation (sight of the naked female body).

working together

- Remember that physical contact does not have to automatically lead to sex. Get into the habit of touching your partner, whether by kissing, cuddling, or stroking and explain to him or her why you are doing this and why it is important that this sort of touching should not always lead to sex.
- Optimize your bodies' ability to respond to sex by looking at the way you live your lives: what you eat, how you sleep, whether or not you smoke, and the amount of alcohol you drink can all play a part.
- Don't put pressure on one another to have sex to make a baby and remember that all sex problems involve both the mind and the body.

- Learn to open up to one another about what you want and like sexually and be prepared to change your sexual style if need be.
- Keep the lines of communication open at all times, both during sex and during everyday life with your partner. Emotions play a vital part in your relationship and, if he or she is not aware of what you are thinking and feeling, your sex life will suffer. If necessary, seek counselling or sex therapy to get to the root of problems.
- There are many good books that can show you how to talk to your partner about sex in a constructive, rather than destructive, way. Your GP may also be able to help, so it is worth discussing the situation with him or her.

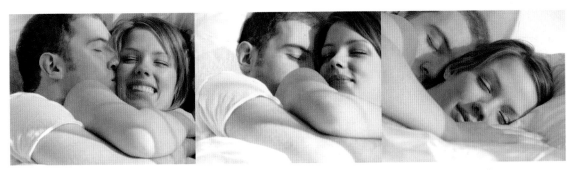

Don't lose sight of why you are with your partner in the first place and make time for physical contact that doesn't lead to sex.

questionnaire: **your sex life**

Sex is likely to be **high on your agenda** right now as you try for a baby, but paradoxically it can be the **part of your relationship that suffers most**. Complete this questionnaire separately, scoring 1 for each "yes" – then compare scores. There are specific **male and female questions at the end**, otherwise most are relevant to you both

1 Has your sex life suffered since you started trying for a baby?
yes ☐ **no** ☐
This is extremely common, especially if you have been trying for a few months.

2 Is sex less adventurous and fun now that you are trying for a baby?
yes ☐ **no** ☐
This may affect your chances of getting pregnant as well as damage your sex life (see page 64).

3 Do you "plan" sex rather than let it happen spontaneously?
yes ☐ **no** ☐
Planning "baby" sex, rather than having sex purely for enjoyment is often detrimental to a couple's sex life.

4 Are you regularly too tired to make love?
yes ☐ **no** ☐
Many couples find that one of the biggest problems they have relating to sex is tiredness. Inevitably, this has a big impact on their chances of getting pregnant.

5 Does it seem like kissing and cuddling always has to lead to sex?
yes ☐ **no** ☐
It is important to be able to touch each other without it leading to sex (see page 73).

 6 Do you tend to limit sex to the time when you (or your partner) is most fertile?
yes ☐ **no** ☐
There is a powerful myth that this increases male potency, but in fact the opposite is true (see page 64).

7 Do you have sex less than twice a week?
yes ☐ **no** ☐
It is important to have sex at least every two to three days during the fertile "window" and regularly during the rest of your cycle (see page 64).

 8 Do you find it harder to get aroused since you started trying for a baby?
yes ☐ **no** ☐
You are probably feeling pressured by the need to achieve a pregnancy and it's affecting your libido. In addition, lack of spontaneity in sex is a big turn-off for men and women alike (see page 64).

 9 Is your relationship suffering since you started trying for a baby?
yes ☐ **no** ☐
Problems with your sex life affect your relationship, and vice versa. When you start trying to get pregnant, it's easy to forget about the other things you enjoy doing as a couple. Make time for them.

10 Do you regularly avoid sex out of frustration, resentment, or anger?

yes ☐ **no** ☐

Try to communicate your feelings more with your partner, rather than miss out on opportunities to have sex. The long-term health of your relationship depends on good communication.

11 Do you find it difficult to talk to your partner about your feelings regarding sex now you are planning a family?

yes ☐ **no** ☐

It is important to keep all channels of communication open to prevent negative emotions setting in (see pages 68–69).

12 (women only) Do you provide your man with lots of details about your menstrual cycle?

yes ☐ **no** ☐

Many men find these details a turn-off. Don't tell him everything (see page 66)!

13 (men only) Are you now an expert on her fertility but wish that you weren't so knowledgeable?

yes ☐ **no** ☐

If checks and treatment are involved, be supportive. But you can ask for these conversations to take place outside the bedroom (see page 66).

14 (women only) Do you expect your man to perform at the drop of a hat?

yes ☐ **no** ☐

Don't be surprised if he can't always perform on demand (see page 66).

15 (men only) Do you feel like a sperm machine, rather than a man who is loved for who he is?

yes ☐ **no** ☐

Find the right time to talk to your partner (preferably in a non-confrontational way). Humour helps.

your**score**

0–3 You generally have a healthy sex life. Although you are trying for a baby, you are still getting a lot of enjoyment out of sex. But you need to ensure that the one or two areas where things aren't ideal don't start to cause problems at a future date.

4–7 You have some problems with your sex life. Some of these – such as frequency of sex – may be quite easy to fix. Others – such as arousal, and the expectation to perform on demand – may require more effort on the part of each of you before they can be resolved.

8–13 You need to address a significant number of issues in your relationship before your sex life deteriorates any further. The risk is that both could suffer permanent damage. Re-read this step and focus on the problem areas that ring true and then try some of the suggested strategies. Communicate your thoughts and emotions with your partner and consider going for some counselling sessions. You need to invest time and effort in improving your sex life if you want your relationship to survive.

step**four**

75

sex and passion

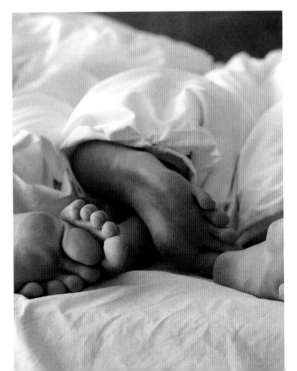

Identify areas of your life where you feel you need to **make adjustments** to improve your **chances of natural conception**

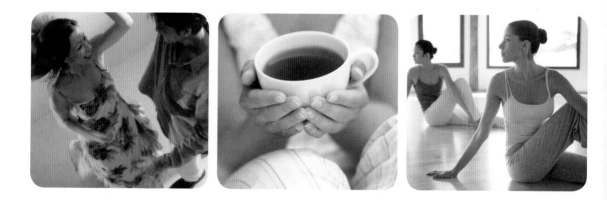

step**five**
lifestyle checks

Your questions answered on:

step five: **lifestyle checks**

Inevitably, the way you **live your life** will have an impact on your fertility: alcohol, cigarettes, excessive stress, exercise (or lack of it), and work can all affect your **chances of conceiving**. This step helps you to assess whether any areas of your life need changing. A good way of doing this is to focus on each **key area** a week at a time

Q Does drinking alcohol impact on fertility?

For both men and women, excessive alcohol intake causes free radicals to flood the body (see page 104), disrupting its proper functioning and damaging egg and sperm production. It also impairs the absorption of essential vitamins and minerals, and zinc.

In men, alcohol damages sperm and affects hormone secretion. It acts directly on the testes, lowering the levels of testosterone and increasing the levels of the female hormone, oestrogen. As a result, sex drive goes down and sperm production (spermatogenesis) is impaired. Excessive alcohol intake is also a common cause of impotence and infertility, and studies have shown that if men drink more than 20 units of alcohol a week (which equates to less than three units per day) it lowers sperm count and increases the incidence of poor motility and morphology (see page 56), and as a result doubles the length of time it takes for their partner to conceive.

Women who have an excessive alcohol intake can suffer from the absence of periods (amenorrhoea – see page 34) or ovulation disorders. In addition, pregnant women who consume more than 14 units a week, particularly during the all-important first trimester (see pages 172–74), have an increased risk of miscarriage, pregnancy complications, and of having a baby with fetal abnormalities.

Q How does alcohol affect blood sugar levels?

Women, in particular, need to keep their blood sugar levels stable in order to balance their hormones and to improve their chances of getting pregnant. Alcohol contains sugars and drinking more than the odd glass of wine or drinking on a daily basis can result in fluctuating blood sugar levels and a craving for more alcohol (see below).

The net result is either that the woman drinks more to keep her blood sugar level raised or she eats sugary foods to raise it. In either case, her health suffers and, in particular, her hormone secretion, which may impact on her fertility.

Q How does the body respond to fluctuating blood sugar levels?

Alcohol raises your blood sugar level, which in turn prompts the secretion of the "feel-good" hormone serotonin. This explains why, when we feel under stress, our bodies sometimes crave alcohol to help us relax. In order to cope with the increase in blood sugar, your body produces large amounts of insulin (a hormone secreted by the pancreas). Insulin allows your body to metabolize the sugar in your blood and move it into your cells to supply energy. As a result, within about 20 to 30 minutes your blood sugar level starts to plummet and the "high" produced by the serotonin starts to diminish, leaving you craving another alcoholic drink. When your blood sugar level drops abruptly and does not go up again, adrenaline is produced to counteract the low glucose level in the blood. This results in mood swings, irritability, and lack of energy. These symptoms are very common in women whose blood sugar levels yo-yo constantly. In addition, their adrenal glands can become exhausted due to the extra demands for adrenaline production and this can have serious consequences for hormone secretion and therefore fertility.

find out more: **how much alcohol?**

In an ideal world, it would be preferable not to drink at all while trying to conceive. However, I am a realist and I know that it can be hard to give up alcohol completely. Moreover, there is no clear evidence that having an occasional glass of wine harms fertility and if this helps reduce your stress levels it could even be beneficial to your chances of conceiving. Consequently, I advise my female clients to drink no more than five units of alcohol a week and men to drink no more than seven. There is some research to say that you shouldn't drink around ovulation, so I encourage clients not to drink at all around this time.

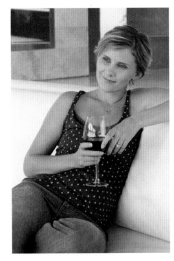

There is no clear evidence that drinking alcohol in moderation has a detrimental effect on fertility.

sensible **drinking**

It is especially important that you pace yourselves, rather than abstaining for several days and then binge drinking throughout an entire evening. It is far better for your body to have to cope with the odd unit of alcohol, rather than having to metabolize an entire week's allowance in just a few hours.

what is a unit of alcohol?

One unit of alcohol is 10ml by volume, or 8g by weight, of pure alcohol. Here are the unit values for alcoholic drinks:

■ Half a pint of ordinary strength beer, lager, or cider (3 to 4 per cent alcohol) is one unit. Strong beer (6 per cent alcohol) contains six units of alcohol in 1 litre (just under 2 pints). One pint is roughly three units.

■ A small glass (125ml) of ordinary strength wine (12 per cent alcohol) equals one and a half units of alcohol. If you drink a third of a bottle of wine (250ml) – two small glasses – you have had three units.
■ A small pub measure (25ml) of spirits (40 per cent alcohol) is one unit. A standard pub measure (35ml) of spirits equals one and a half units of alcohol.

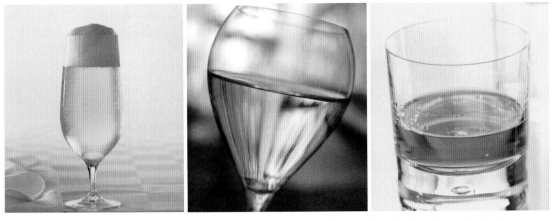

Be aware that strong continental lagers can have a high alcohol content.

Choose a standard-sized glass of wine rather than the large ones many pubs offer.

Don't be tempted by the double measures of spirits on offer during pub happy hours.

Q I am a smoker. How will this affect my chances of conceiving?

The evidence that cigarettes directly harm female fertility is unequivocal. There are many substances found in cigarettes, including cadmium, lead, and nicotine, which are toxic (not to mention carcinogenic) and are thought to have a harmful effect on the endometrium (the lining of the uterus) and on ovarian function. Smoking also depletes the body's reserves of certain important vitamins and minerals, notably zinc, selenium, and vitamin C. Smoking has been linked to poor cervical mucus and is known to affect the endocrine system, which regulates hormonal secretion.

Studies have shown that female smokers have a 40 per cent lower chance of getting pregnant. Smoking accelerates the loss of eggs and damage to DNA. As a result, eggs either cannot be fertilized or they miscarry soon after implantation. Finally, smoking can knock as many as 10 years off your reproductive life and you may reach the menopause much earlier than you would have done if you were a non-smoker.

Q Do **recreational drugs** affect fertility?

Whatever you may believe, there are no "safe" recreational drugs to use when you are trying to conceive, nor "safe" levels at which you can take them. All recreational drugs have an effect on fertility, either because they damage sperm production or because they affect male and/or female hormone production. Furthermore, while the effects of drugs on your metabolism are reversible, it may take a few months (and in some cases, years) for this to happen, during which time you may become pregnant, and your unborn child may suffer from the effects of the drugs that are still in your system. If you are an occasional user of recreational drugs, stop now. If you are drug-dependent, you will need to seek professional help to ensure that you give up as quickly as possible, and to give yourself the best chance of conceiving a healthy child.

Marijuana Smoking cannabis is damaging to male fertility in particular. One of its principal active ingredients, tetrahydrocannabinol (THC), is chemically related to testosterone and even when taken in small quantities, it lowers testosterone levels, decreases the volume of seminal fluid, damages sperm motility, and causes increased numbers of abnormal sperm and a lower sperm count. As it also lowers libido, it is hardly conducive to having a good sex life!

In women, cannabis can have a toxic effect on the developing egg and disrupts ovulation. Women who smoke the drug also secrete small amounts of THC into their vaginal fluid. Sperm that come into contact with this absorb the drug and their motility is affected.

Cocaine, opiates, and ecstasy These drugs have all been shown to have dramatic effects on both male and female fertility. Men who take these drugs often suffer from reduced libido, abnormally shaped sperm, and poor sperm count. There is also an increased risk of genetic problems in the sperm. Women who take them often suffer from ovulatory problems, menstrual irregularities, and reduced ovarian reserve and there is a known link between babies born with birth defects and the use of these drugs. Cocaine damages the functioning of the fallopian tubes and significantly increases the risk of miscarriage. This drug also crosses the placenta and affects the baby in the uterus. He or she may be born drug-dependent, and suffer from serious withdrawal symptoms and possible brain damage.

Anabolic steroids Recreational body-builders (invariably men) who take anabolic steroids will suffer very clear and severe side effects within a short space of time, as these drugs affect hormone production. Consequently, testicular function is affected and, within a few months, sperm production is severely reduced and often ceases altogether. Motility and morphology are also damaged (see page 56). Decreased libido is also a known side effect. It can take anything from 12 months to three years for the effects of anabolic steroids to be reversed.

Q My partner smokes regularly. Does he have to stop too?

Men who smoke have a 30 to 70 per cent lower sperm count than men who are non-smokers. They also have increased abnormalities in sperm shape and function and poorer motility. Male smoking is also thought to be responsible for up to 120,000 cases of impotence every year in men aged 30 to 50 years old. Male smoking is therefore a strong factor in reducing a couple's overall chances of conceiving.

Q How long does it take for fertility to improve if I stop smoking?

Research has indicated that, within a year of stopping smoking, ex-smokers take no longer to become pregnant than those who have never smoked. Even two months after they had stopped smoking, couples who were attempting IVF significantly improved their chances of conceiving.

Q How does smoking affect the chances of success with IVF treatment?

Women who are undergoing IVF treatment and who smoke need nearly twice as many attempts to conceive as non-smoking women. They need higher doses of ovary-stimulating gonadotrophins, and fewer eggs are retrieved and fertilized. They also have a higher miscarriage rate than non-smokers. Moreover, a Canadian study has shown that the odds of a woman conceiving are improved only minimally if it is her partner rather than she who smokes: they are still roughly half those of non-smokers. In other words, it doesn't matter whether it is the man or the woman who smokes: IVF and smoking do not mix!

Q Why is smoking harmful once conception has taken place?

Once you conceive, if you are a smoker you have double the risk of miscarriage because smoking directly affects blood flow to the uterus. According to one recent BMA study, smoking and passive smoking are responsible for up to 5,000 miscarriages a year. In addition, because smoking prevents the placenta from receiving the maximum amount of blood supply, and therefore oxygen, it may not function properly and the growth of the fetus may be impeded. As a result, women who smoke have a 50 per cent increase in the risk of premature birth, and twice the chance of having a low-birth-weight baby, with all the complications that this brings.

Smoking also affects the cilia (microscopic hair-like projections) lining the fallopian tubes, so smokers are at higher risk of an ectopic pregnancy (see page 26) as the rate of progress made by the fertilized egg along the tubes can be reduced.

A pregnant woman who smokes has a much greater risk of developing serious pregnancy complications such as pre-eclampsia (with symptoms of high blood pressure and swelling of feet, legs, and hands) and placental abruptions (where the placenta separates from the lining of the uterus, depriving the fetus of oxygen).

There is also evidence that smoking increases the incidence of fetal malformations such as cleft palate. Perinatal death (stillbirth and death within the first year of life) is also much higher among the babies of women who smoke.

Q How can I stop smoking?

There is absolutely no valid reason why you should continue to smoke while you are trying to conceive. And given that the benefits start to show within two months of stopping, it seems clear that, if you smoke, you should stop today and do everything possible to ensure that you stop for good. Cognitive behaviour therapy (CBT), which aims to change patterns of thinking or behaviour (see page 137), and hypnotherapy (see page 133) are among the many very effective programmes that can help smokers to give up. GP practices often run clinics that help people to stop smoking, so ask your GP or practice nurse for details. Aids such as nicotine patches and gum are also available from pharmacies or through your GP.

> ### Zita's **tip**
> Make sure you both **give up smoking** and don't be afraid to **ask for help**!

Q Why do we get stressed?

Stress often arises because we do not feel in control of a particular area of our lives. If your work is going well or your finances are healthy, the chances are they are not causing you any stress. However, if you rarely take a holiday or are constantly short of sleep because you are worrying about work or debts, you will probably have raised levels of stress hormones.

Stress levels often rise when couples start trying for a baby. There is no doubt that trying and failing to get pregnant month after month does also impact on levels of stress which, in turn, can affect a woman's fertility. I see many women who are highly able, organized people, used to planning every area of their lives and to reaping the rewards of hard work and dedication. Suddenly, they start trying to get pregnant and realize that their fertility, which up until now they had controlled (by actively avoiding getting

find out more: **responding to stress**

The body is primed to deal with physical threats and stresses with a rapid set of defences known as the "fight or flight" response. However, problems occur when these high-gear reactions occur in response to psychological stressors too – anything from managing a huge workload to making ends meet. Triggered repeatedly these inevitably take their toll on the body.

The nervous system is a vast network of nerves that branch out from the brain and spinal cord to reach every part of the body; it is the source of our consciousness and the initiator of all our actions. It also has autonomic functions that monitor and control the body's internal environment and unconscious processes such as breathing. The working partners within the autonomic nervous system are the sympathetic and the parasympathetic branches, which have opposing effects but balance each other most of the time. The sympathetic branch helps us respond to an emergency, and deal with stress, frustration, and anger by speeding up thinking and getting us prepared for action (see below). The parasympathetic branch restores a resting state that is important to well-being and fertility.

psychological **stress factors**

- major life changes, illness, or the death of a loved one
- not being able to achieve a goal (such as having a child)
- troubled interpersonal relationships, work, and money worries
- anxiety about global and local issues in the papers and on TV.

responses of the autonomic nervous system		
body part	**sympathetic response**	**parasympathetic response**
Eyes	Pupils dilate to sharpen vision.	Pupils constrict and vision returns to normal.
Lungs	Bronchial tubes dilate to boost oxygen intake.	Bronchial tubes constrict and breathing returns to normal.
Heart	Rate and strength of heartbeat increase and blood reaches muscles faster.	Rate and strength of heartbeat return to normal.
Stomach	Enzyme production decreases and digestion slows.	Enzyme production returns to normal.
Liver	Releases glucose and boosts energy.	Stores glucose.

pregnant), is largely beyond their control. This comes as a shock and affects them deeply, although not always consciously at first, and their stress hormone levels rise.

Q Does stress affect fertility?

Nearly everyone has some form of stress in their lives. Where people differ is in their response to stress and the levels of stress hormones produced as a result. When a woman's body starts to secrete excessive amounts of stress hormones, these interfere with the secretion of the female sex hormones, and, in some women, menstruation and ovulation disruption can follow, which then leads to difficulty with conception (see page 84).

What is also clear is that stress often affects a couple's social life, sex life, and general happiness, which can cause reduced libido in the male or female partner (or both) and that inevitably affects their chances of getting pregnant.

living life with alarm bells ringing

During life's difficult moments the hypothalamus in the brain triggers a sequence of nervous and hormonal signals that prompt the adrenal glands to release a surge of hormones, the most abundant being cortisol and adrenaline. Cortisol increases the level of glucose in the bloodstream and enhances the brain's use of glucose. It also has a shutting-down effect on less essential functions such as digestion and reproduction. Meanwhile adrenaline increases the heart rate, elevates blood pressure, and boosts energy to prime the body for action.

The result is a pounding heart, fast breathing, and rapid sweat release – useful if you have to flee or fight but inappropriate in response to a tight deadline or demanding email at work. What is more, modern stresses tend to be prolonged and the body can end up on red alert for longer than it should be. Overproduction of stress hormones, especially cortisol, can exhaust the adrenal glands (see page 84). Overexposure to these hormones can also disrupt many body processes, increasing the risk of obesity, insomnia, digestive and fertility problems, heart disease, and depression.

The hypothalamus responds to stress signals passed on from other areas of the brain by relaying the message to the pituitary gland

The pituitary gland then secretes ACTH, a hormone that in turn tells the adrenal glands to start producing stress hormones, including cortisol and adrenaline

Cortisol and adrenaline are released as part of a complex alarm system that affects heart rate and breathing and regions of the brain that control mood, motivation, and fear

ACTH

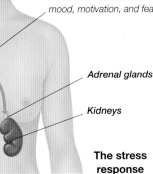

Adrenal glands

Kidneys

The stress response

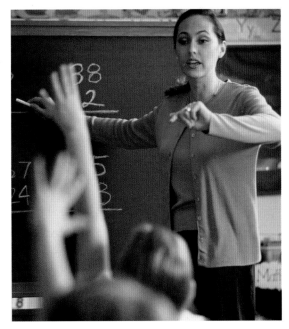

Stress is common in modern life, but people vary in their sensitivity to it and can learn strategies to control their response.

Q Does stress have effects on female hormones?

As well as regulating stress hormones, the hypothalamus in the brain controls the sex hormones of the female reproductive cycle by producing gonadotrophin-releasing hormone (GnRH) at the beginning of the menstrual cycle. This tells the pituitary gland to release follicle-stimulating hormone (FSH), which in turn stimulates the production of oestrogen, luteinizing hormone (LH), and progesterone at specific times in the menstrual cycle. At times of severe stress, or when a woman suffers from chronic stress, progesterone may be converted to the stress hormone cortisol, which is produced along the same biochemical pathways as the sex hormones. The result is a decrease in the levels of progesterone in the body. At the same time, levels of prolactin, a hormone produced by the pituitary gland, stay raised, due to decreased amounts of the feel-good hormone dopamine, and this results in a decrease in the normal level of sex hormones. Whenever the secretion of any of these sex hormones is affected, ovulatory and menstrual problems may occur.

Q How does stress affect digestion?

When adrenaline is released into the bloodstream, glucose is released to give the body the energy it needs to prepare for the "fight or flight" response (see page 82). If you are able to recover from the surge of adrenaline, your body's blood sugar levels can return to normal. If you cannot, because your adrenaline and cortisol levels are constantly raised, your adrenal glands start to suffer from exhaustion. At that stage, you may begin to experience symptoms such as poor digestion, reduced ability to absorb nutrients, and even food allergies, caused by prolonged exposure to stress.

Q How can I cope better with stress?

It is not possible to eliminate all stress from our lives, nor is it desirable to do so – a small degree of stress keeps our bodies primed and our brains challenged and sharp. However, it is important to prevent stress from damaging our physiological and psychological well-being.

The way in which you cope with stress, both as a couple and as an individual, will determine whether or not it continues to have a harmful effect. Your management of stress depends on various factors, including your personality, your upbringing, previous stressful experiences and outcomes, and how much support you have received. Understanding stress, understanding how you have reacted to it in the past, and assessing whether you need to change your reaction, are vital prior to conceiving and especially if you have fertility problems or are undergoing IVF treatment. This will also give you the feeling that you have regained control over your emotions and you will feel calmer as a result.

Being able to analyse which areas of your life need addressing in order to reduce stress and learning how to relax are the two key ways in which you can alter your mood, balance your hormones, and improve your general health. The consequence will be an improvement in your chances of conceiving.

Chinese medicine believes in building up your reserves so that you can cope with difficult situations in life. And I believe that you need to build up those reserves by leading a healthy lifestyle, having sufficient sleep and a good diet, taking regular exercise, and using relaxation techniques.

Emotions such as frustration, anxiety, resentment, and conflict all cause stress responses in our bodies. Learning to manage those emotions is key to our mental and physical health and will determine the extent to which they affect us.

Your fertility depends very much on the good functioning of your endocrine system. By understanding how your lifestyle or diet contribute to your stress levels and to your hormonal balance, you can find ways of making the changes you need in order to maximize your chances of conceiving. Step 7 discusses various ways of managing stress, including relaxation and visualization techniques.

Q Why is sleep so important?

All the physiological cycles of our bodies are regulated by the sleep–wake cycle, and the more it is disrupted, the more they will be affected. At night, our bodies repair tissue, enabling us to heal more quickly, and our conscious brain activity is switched off, which is essential if we are to feel alert the next day. Our corticosteroid levels and our temperature drop, and both rise again in the morning, which is why we often feel cold if we have to get up in the middle of the night. Our immune system and hormone secretion also vary according to whether it is day or night-time, and levels of the hormone melatonin (the only hormone to be secreted by the pineal gland – a small gland deep in the brain), rise at night and fall again during the day (see page 86). Melatonin, which is a derivative of the mood-influencing hormone serotonin, is responsible for maintaining our day–night balance. It is the secretion of melatonin as darkness falls that makes us feel sleepy.

Hormone imbalance due to lack of sleep can also lead to menstrual irregularity, making it harder to conceive.

Q I'm often too tired for sex. How can I improve the situation?

On a very practical level, a good amount of sleep is essential in order to feel energized. Many of the couples I see don't seem to have much stamina. While they might just about get through the day, by the evening they are flagging, and the net result is that they are simply too tired to have sex. Alternatively, some of them go to bed very late, by which time they are too exhausted and too tired for sex. Either way, these couples waste valuable opportunities for conception by having inadequate amounts of sleep or poor sleeping habits.

If you find you are often too tired for sex, you need to look at how much sleep you are getting and find ways of going to bed earlier. Don't go to the other extreme and bring your bedtime forward by an entire hour, for example, as your body clock will have trouble readjusting (see pages 86–87). Instead, make the change gradually, going to bed 15 minutes earlier one week, then another 15 minutes the next, until you feel you have found the

right time for you: you should not be overly tired and you should be able to have sex if you want to. If not, you should be able to slip easily into a relaxed state that brings on sleep soon afterwards.

Q What's the best way to make sure I get a good night's sleep?

There are lots of things you can do to help ensure you get a good night's sleep:

■ Don't work too late or pay your bills last thing at night. It takes time for your brain to switch off, and you will find yourself taking your anxieties to bed with you. The same applies to watching TV – try reading a book instead.

■ Try to to have your last meal or snack at least two hours before going to bed and don't eat a heavy evening meal. Your digestion and your sleep will improve as a result. Don't drink alcohol, caffeinated drinks, or drinks that are high in vitamin C (such as orange juice) in the evening, as they are stimulants and will stop you going to sleep. Drink a herbal tea, such as camomile.

■ Women should have a relaxing bath in a softly lit bathroom. Men, however, should avoid this, as long hot baths will raise the temperature of their testes and this will not help sperm production.

■ Try to go to bed at a similar time every night, and to get up at a similar time every day, weekends included. Keep your bedroom dark and quiet. Don't toss and turn for hours in bed. If you can't sleep, try tensing and then relaxing all the muscles in your body, starting from the toes and working up. If you still can't sleep, get up, have a hot drink, such as hot milk or camomile tea, to relax you, and read a book.

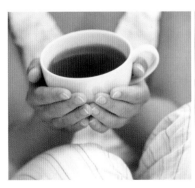

Herbal teas such as camomile have a recognized sleep-inducing effect.

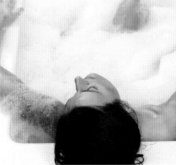

Relaxation is key to being able to sleep – enjoy a hot soak before you go to bed.

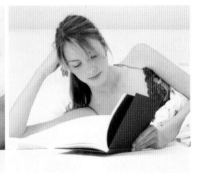

If you can't sleep, don't toss and turn for hours. Try reading a book for a while.

find out more: **circadian rhythm**

Our bodies have evolved to co-ordinate activity with the day–night cycle caused by the Earth's rotation, in a pattern known as our circadian rhythm.

The word "circadian" comes from the Latin words *circa* and *dian* meaning, literally, "about a day". In fact, our natural body clock runs on slightly longer than a 24-hour day – it is nearer 25 hours. But it resets itself on a daily basis thanks to daylight stimulating the retina and the body's internal biological clock, which is controlled by the hypothalamus in the brain. This is why the body runs on "local" time, and why it cannot adjust immediately if there is a change in the day–night pattern – when we travel across time zones, for example.

70% of people don't get **enough sleep**

Sleep is integral to our quality of life, our health, and our fertility. On average, we need eight hours' sleep a night but rarely seem to get it.

changing with **the seasons**

- During wintertime we need more sleep. Many mammals hibernate and most people find it hard to get out of bed when it is still dark outside.
- In summer, people tend to wake naturally and may not need an alarm clock.
- IVF and ICSI cycles are more successful in the summer when daylight lasts longer than during the darker winter months. This may be related to the effects of melatonin (see page 85).

our daily highs and lows

Our circadian rhythm also means that during the day there are times when we are more energetic than others. Some people are more conscious of this than others, but, for example, many people are aware of the "graveyard slot" in public speaking, which is straight after lunch when audiences are often not very alert. Usually, people are at their most productive in the morning, until around 1pm. Between 3 and 5pm there is often a dip in energy, and indeed in many cultures people have a siesta during those hours. Between about 5 and 8pm, many people have a second burst of productivity, and, in fact, if they were asked to go to sleep during those hours they would find it extremely difficult to do so, whereas they would easily have managed a post-lunch nap just a couple of hours earlier. After 8pm, the body's metabolism begins to slow down naturally and levels of the hormone melatonin begin to climb in readiness for sleep.

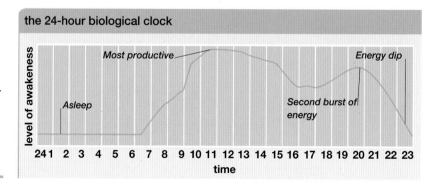

the 24-hour biological clock

level of awakeness

Most productive

Energy dip

Asleep

Second burst of energy

24 1 2 3 4 5 6 7 8 9 10 11 12 13 14 15 16 17 18 19 20 21 22 23

time

a good night's sleep

While much of the body rests during sleep, the nerve cells in the brain continue to send signals and these can be picked up on EEG traces. These traces reveal different waveforms of brain activity for each of five stages of sleep (see below). These are made up of lengthening phases of rapid eye movement (REM) sleep, when dreaming occurs, and four stages of deeper non-rapid eye movement (NREM) sleep, which is dreamless. As the body reaches the deeper stages, temperature, heartbeat rate, breathing rate, and blood pressure all reduce. When we go to sleep we move quickly into a deep, restorative sleep, then come back up towards wakefulness, then go back down again. One full sleep cycle takes about 90 minutes and research shows that we get our important "core" sleep in about six hours.

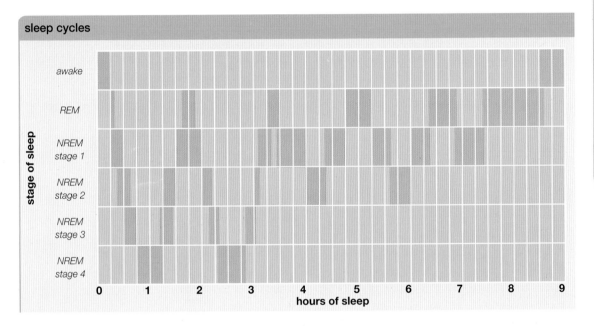

sleep cycles

weekend disruption

Disruption of the body clock and sleep can happen simply because people go to bed much later at the weekend than they do during the week and get up later as a result on Saturday and Sunday mornings. They then find it frustrating and stressful that on Sunday night they cannot get to sleep, and on Monday morning they feel exhausted. This is because by Sunday evening their body clock is all over the place: it has just about adapted to getting up late that morning, and it is now being asked to readjust to the earlier bedtimes of weekdays. When you add to this the fact that people can be a bit anxious on Sunday night about the week ahead, it is no surprise to discover that, for many of us, we start our working week having had the worst night's sleep of the entire seven days.

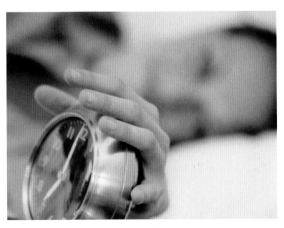

If you go to bed or get up at very different times from one day to the next, your biological clock will have trouble adjusting.

Q Is exercise important to fertility?

Regular exercise is definitely recommended for fertility and as a preparation for pregnancy. It only becomes harmful to your chances of conception if you are exercising so vigorously and so frequently that it affects your hormones, your menstrual cycle, and even your immune system (see page 89). Unless you have had more than two consecutive miscarriages or are undergoing IVF treatment – in which case you should check with your doctor about how much and when to exercise – I would not advise anyone to stop exercising. It is also fine to exercise through the time when you ovulate and during the last two weeks of your cycle when an embryo might be in the very early stages of implantation. There is no evidence to suggest that women should cut out exercise during these times if they are already used to a certain level.

Q What are the best forms of exercise?

There is no such thing as good and bad exercise when it comes to helping your chances of conceiving. I always advise clients to try a range of different types, so that they are less likely to get bored by what they are doing. That is also the best way to ensure that their body benefits as much as possible, as different forms of exercise use different muscles and have varying effects.

Broadly speaking, there are two forms of exercise: aerobic and anaerobic, and ideally you should do both for maximum health benefits. Aerobic means "with oxygen" and can be defined as any activity that works the larger muscle groups and the lungs and raises the heart rate. The activity needs to be maintained at a moderate intensity for a long duration. Typical aerobic activities include walking, running, cycling, and swimming.

Anaerobic exercise means "without oxygen" and comprises brief, strength-based activities where the muscles are required to work hard in short bursts. Sprinting, weight-training, and jumping are all anaerobic forms of exercise.

Many sports are a combination of both: tennis, badminton, skiing, and football, for example, involve bursts of sprinting or intense demands on certain muscles, but they also make longer, more continuous demands on the heart, lungs, and large muscle groups. Activities such as yoga and pilates are excellent for strengthening and toning, breathing correctly, and releasing tension.

If you are not used to exercising regularly, avoid launching yourself into a gruelling fitness regime from day one. Start with, for example, swimming, brisk walking, or cycling for 20 minutes three times a week.

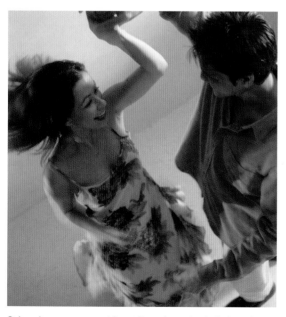

Salsa classes are a great form of exercise: not only do they give you a sustained aerobic workout, they are fun to try together.

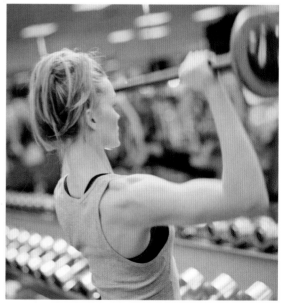

Weight-training is an anaerobic form of exercise. Make sure you ask for some supervision if you are new to this particular activity.

Q How does **exercise** help fertility?

Irrespective of whether or not you are trying to get pregnant, exercise is good for your overall health, and this is likely to impact on your fertility.

It produces endorphins Mood-boosting endorphins, biochemical compounds, are produced by the pituitary gland in response to aerobic exercise. Because endorphins reduce pain and give a sense of well-being, they are often referred to as the body's "natural painkillers". If you exercise regularly, you will notice that you feel energized and optimistic after a good workout, even if you were tired and lethargic before starting. This improves your chances of getting pregnant as you will have more energy for sex.

It relieves stress When endorphins are racing around your bloodstream after exercise, they lower stress levels and give you a sense of elation. This feeling can last several hours, if not all day, and the more this happens regularly, the more your stress will be reduced on a permanent basis, and that will be good for your fertility (see page 82).

It helps digestion The fact that you move around much more when you exercise significantly reduces digestive problems, such as constipation and the bloating and poor digestion that can accompany a sluggish intestine. If food passes through you more quickly you will feel better, and are less likely to suffer from heartburn and indigestion. That said, avoid exercising just after a meal because while you are digesting, blood flow is concentrated in the stomach. Exercise will disrupt the process and may make you feel light-headed.

It controls blood sugar Exercise helps keep your blood sugar levels stable, because insulin secretion (from the pancreas) is more effective during bouts of physical activity. Regular exercise increases the number of insulin receptors in your cells. Insulin attaches to these receptors so that sugar can pass from the blood into other cells in the body. Having more receptors makes the body more sensitive to insulin and, as a result, insulin works more efficiently and you will need less of it.

Of course, the release of adrenaline during exercise also causes blood sugar levels to rise temporarily, as sugar (in the form of glycogen) is released from the stores in the muscles and liver. But in this situation you will not get the blood sugar high and then the ensuing crash that you might get when you eat sugary foods, for example. There will be a more gradual readjustment of blood sugar levels. And the fitter you are, the slower the drop will be.

It is good for blood flow Exercise increases lung capacity and builds up heart muscle, as well as other muscles, and this enables blood to be pumped round the body more effectively. As a result, every part of your body is well supplied with nutrients and oxygen in the blood, and uses them more efficiently; and waste product from dead or damaged cells is eliminated. In this way, your body regenerates itself and heals more quickly. Exercise does not put a strain on your body's systems. On the contrary, it makes them work better and more easily, and that can only be good for your overall health and good for your fertility.

It is good for weight management Whether you do aerobic or anaerobic exercise, you will work your muscles and raise your heart rate, and this will burn calories and help control weight, even if you are eating the same amount as you normally do. This is a wonderful way of avoiding the yo-yo dieting that so many women experience. Your weight loss is more likely to be permanent and your health improved on a long-term basis.

It helps the immune system Moderate exercise has been shown to improve the positive immune system response and to boost the production of cells that attack bacteria. Consequently, regular exercise can lead to substantial benefits in the immune system's well-being. It is worth noting, however, that excessive, intense exercise has the opposite effect on the immune system because the body then produces excessive amounts of the stress hormones cortisol and adrenaline, and these raise blood pressure and cholesterol levels and suppress the immune system.

find out more: **how much exercise?**

Ideally, you should be doing 30 minutes of aerobic exercise three times a week, and some resistance exercise such as gym work twice a week. I'm realistic enough, however, to know that this might not be possible for a lot of people. Exercising three times a week in some shape or form, and for a minimum of 20 minutes, will still improve your level of fitness and stamina, tone your muscles, and benefit your health in general. The exercise you do should be of moderate intensity. As a rule of thumb, this means that it makes you a little warm and sweaty, and slightly out of breath as your heart and breathing rates increase.

Whatever forms of exercise you choose, try to find activities that you enjoy and then do them on a regular basis to make the most of your good intentions. It doesn't matter whether you do a modern dance class, join a gym, or go riding – as long as you enjoy your exercise, you are more likely to want to keep it up. We have all started a new activity with the best of intentions, then given up after only a few weeks because it doesn't really fit in with our lives. Before you begin, think carefully about what you choose to do.

66%
of adults do not **exercise regularly**

Bear in mind that walking to the next tube or bus stop on your way to work or climbing stairs rather than using a lift or even doing some vigorous housework can each count as one of your weekly activities.

taking **care**

- ▪ Avoid exercising to exhaustion.
- ▪ Avoid overheating from excessive exercise or from saunas or steam rooms (this is also important for men).
- ▪ Keep your weight/BMI within normal limits (see page 13).
- ▪ If you think reducing your exercise regime would be difficult to achieve, you could be overdoing it. As ever, it is a question of keeping the right balance.

create your own exercise plan

I believe that if you make a plan of what exercise you will do, you can devise a regime that can really work for you and your lifestyle.

- ▪ Write down the activities that you already do and how long you do them for each week.
- ▪ Write down all the activities that you would like to start.
- ▪ Assess which ones fall into aerobic or anaerobic exercise, or a mixture of the two.
- ▪ Decide which ones you are going to do and how often. Make sure you are realistic and that your plan fits in with your work, lifestyle, and where you live.
- ▪ Find out how to take up any that you would like to try.
- ▪ Set yourself a target date of when you will start. Book up lessons or classes.

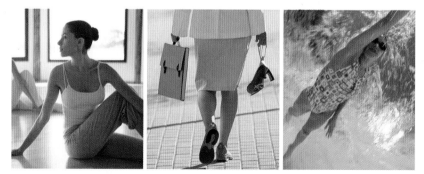

Choose types of exercise that you enjoy and that fit into your lifestyle and daily routine.

Q Can working too hard affect fertility?

I see many couples who work very long hours and are permanently exhausted and under considerable strain as a result. As explained earlier in this step, poor sleep, excessive production of stress hormones, lack of exercise (caused by working very long hours), and poor diet are all detrimental to fertility. So I have no doubt that work can also affect a couple's chances of having a baby, depending on the pressure they are under.

One study showed that women under stress at work had shorter cycles. Their follicular phase was shorter (see page 36), so ovulation was occurring earlier and couples were often not having sex early enough in the cycle to conceive.

If work dominates your life – you don't take all your holidays, work long hours and at weekends, and make work-related phone calls or check e-mails at home – you need to rethink your work–life balance (see page 92).

Q How can I make up my mind whether or not to change my job?

If you think your job is damaging your health and therefore your chances of conceiving, you need to take stock and see what options are open to you. Ask yourself some of the following questions:
- Why am I still in my job?
- Does it pay well (including benefits/pensions)?
- Does it have good maternity/paternity leave provision? (This is often the key work benefit that women don't want/cannot afford to lose).
- Is it a family-friendly company?
- Do the working conditions suit me?
- Is it good for my career progression?
- Where do I see myself professionally in five years' time?

If you feel your job is worth sticking with despite the stress, the next step is to talk to your managers or human resources department about reducing your workload.

Q Our finances are a mess – what can we do to sort them out?

Surveys regularly point to the fact that one of the main subjects that couples argue about is money. It goes without saying that couples with financial worries are likely to be under more strain than people who are free of them. But when a couple is suddenly faced with the prospect of large bills for fertility treatment, for example, they can often become weighed down with the additional burden. This is particularly heavy to bear when they are struggling already to cope with the many physical and psychological difficulties that fertility treatment causes.

Whatever your situation, if money is a worry it is always helpful to sit down and make a detailed list of outgoings and incoming money. If you have pooled your finances in the last few years with your partner, you might never have got round to analysing what comes in, what goes out, and what you can afford each month. In all likelihood, forcing yourselves to look at what money you have at your disposal will actually show you that savings can be made in several ways.

It might also be helpful to speak to a professional about organizing your finances, if only to feel a bit more in control of the situation. As ever, when you gain control, you often gain a sense of renewed calm as well. You feel you are doing something positive to help yourself. And the knock-on effect for your physical and mental health will be apparent in a short space of time.

Q I hate wasting time – what's the point of doing things purely for pleasure?

Many of my clients, both male and female, have so many work and social commitments that they rarely get time on their own, simply to wind down. Yet it is very important for you to have regular time to yourself. A three-day break somewhere idyllic is all very well, but what is equally vital to your long-term well-being – and hence your fertility – is that you programme in, every week if possible, a session of self-indulgence.

To find out if you need to make more time for yourself, think through the following points. Which activities/pastimes/beauty treatments/complementary therapies do you currently do on your own and for pleasure and how often do you do them? Which additional ones would you like to do and how often? How much do they cost? Then identify times/days of the week when they could be fitted in. Set a start date. Be realistic, both financially and in terms of time. It destroys the point if you start getting stressed by an unrealistic timetable!

Remember also that making time for yourself can include going for a walk, shutting yourself in a room with a good book, soaking in a bath, or even doing nothing. It does not have to cost anything or involve you leaving the house. It simply means thinking of yourself and no one else.

Q Are there any good strategies to help me rebalance my life?

To get a clearer idea of whether you have the right balance in your life, draw a pie chart, similar to the ones shown below. Assess what percentage of your time you spend doing each element during a typical week (the areas below are suggestions only). Once you have drawn up your pie chart, you can decide whether you think the balance is right. If it is not, aim to re-adjust the areas that most need work on and that can be changed.

Q How can we make the most of the time we spend together?

It is easy, when you live with someone, to get on a treadmill of routine and rarely venture off it into an activity that you do not normally do together. Yet doing something different invariably has an instant effect of revitalizing the relationship and of placing you both in a situation of novelty and of newly (re)discovered fun. Boredom and familiarity often decrease the amount of pleasure that you get out of each other's company. Think of the first time you

went shopping with your partner, even to the supermarket: the novelty factor of discovering each other's likes and dislikes made the whole experience (almost!) enjoyable. Yet, before long, the whole process becomes a mundane chore. Every couple can benefit from re-injecting that breath of fresh air into their daily lives. It's a question of deciding where that fresh air will come from.

One of the recurring problems that couples complain about is their lack of time. It is true that many of them lack the time to do anything but eat, sleep, and work, but they have to reach a stage where they want to change their lifestyle so that their health, their relationship, and even their fertility improve.

If you always seem to be chronically short of time, then think again: try keeping a diary of everything you do for a week, and the hours at which you do it. Is there any room for manoeuvre? Do you have to work those hours every day? Do you have to spend so long on the shopping, or would it be more time-efficient to buy more of it locally or to shop online? Making a few small time-savings could enable you to take time out with your partner. This might mean a trip to the bowling alley or a walk in the park instead of a walk round the aisles of a supermarket.

Life balance pie charts

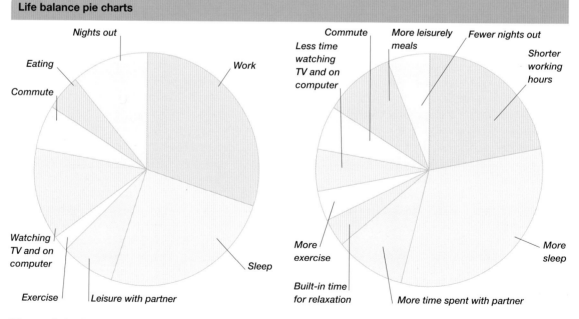

When work dominates your life and all you can do when you get home is to slump in front of the television, there is little time left for leisure activities that make for a healthy lifestyle and improve fertility.

Making slight adjustments to your life balance – increasing time spent exercising and relaxing, for example – will help you improve your health and therefore your chances of conceiving.

Q Should we plan what we do together?

Spend time drawing up a list of which areas or activities you do together that you enjoy. Add to the list any activities, however unlikely, that you would like to do with your partner. Each of you should make your own list, then compare results at the end. There are likely to be a few surprises. Whether these are good or bad, try to be honest with each other without being hurtful, and you will find out a great deal about your partner's likes and dislikes.

The long-term health of your relationship depends on you communicating as well as possible, and this includes talking about your everyday lives and how you spend time together. This will avoid resentment and boredom settling in, which is invariably a passion-killer between two people, and leads to bad or non-existent sex: not good if you are trying to make a baby!

Q Does it matter that we find it really hard to fit in holidays?

I am always surprised by the number of clients I see who do not seem able to take all their annual holiday entitlement. I tell them that, even if they do not go anywhere during their time off, they must at least make sure that they take all the days' leave they can in any given year. Having a mental and physical break from office routine, if only for a couple of days, does wonders for people's mood and energy levels. I also advise them that, once they get back from one holiday, they should try to book ahead for their next break, so that they always have something to look forward to, and they know when they will next be leaving their desk for a while.

Q Are people more fertile on holiday?

I have lost count of the number of couples I have heard about or treated because they were having problems getting pregnant and who returned from holiday, only to discover that they were expecting a baby. It will always be difficult to prove by scientific means that holidays can be a fertile time for couples, but the fact remains that anecdotal evidence does indicate this to be the case. I have no doubt that there is a strong mind–body link whereby couples are relaxed without everyday pressures, and are leading healthier lives. They also are much more likely to have time on their hands and to be having more carefree or passionate sex – for the vast majority of couples, the only missing ingredient for conception is time and opportunity for sex.

Q Are short breaks or long breaks better for health and fertility?

As there is only anecdotal evidence concerning the possible effect that taking a holiday has on a couple's fertility, it is not possible to say what type of holiday is best. Several short breaks might suit some couples better, while others need longer to wind down and relax and might prefer a one- or two-week break. The point of a holiday is that it should focus on your relationship, give you relaxed time together, time to have a lot of sex if possible, and to ensure that your relationship continues to benefit once you return home. Plan your next break, if only as a reward for all the effort you have been making trying to assess and change your lifestyle in order to improve your chances of getting pregnant.

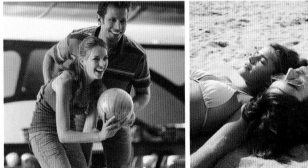

Spending time doing activities you enjoy together can revitalize your relationship.

Holidays can often result in pregnancy even if couples have been having problems.

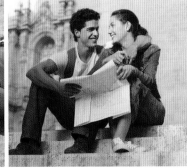

A short break in a foreign city can help put the romance back into your lives.

questionnaire: **balancing lifestyle**

Your **lifestyle cannot be ignored** when you consider the factors that may affect your fertility. Having read this step you will no doubt be aware of at least one **area** you could **improve upon**.
Score 1 for every "yes" answer you give to these questions to find out what your score reveals about the **way you live** your life

1 Do you drink more than 5 units of alcohol a week (if you are a woman) or 7 units (if you are a man)?
yes ☐ **no** ☐
A few units of alcohol will not harm your fertility, but more than this could become a problem (see pages 78–79).

2 Do you drink most of your unit quota in just one or two nights?
yes ☐ **no** ☐
It is much better for your metabolism to pace yourself when it comes to alcohol intake, however low it is.

3 Do you or your partner take recreational drugs?
yes ☐ **no** ☐
There is no safe amount or safe drug that you can take when you are trying to get pregnant (see page 80).

4 Do you or your partner smoke?
yes ☐ **no** ☐
Smoking and babies do not mix! Read pages 80–81 if you are unconvinced.

5 Do you cook a proper meal less than three times a week?
yes ☐ **no** ☐
This is often related to a hectic lifestyle and may also suggest your diet is poor (see Step 6).

6 Do you crave sugary foods on a daily basis?
yes ☐ **no** ☐
The highs and lows caused by blood sugar variations may disrupt hormone balance and can affect fertility (see page 78).

7 Do you often find it hard to fall asleep or to get back to sleep if you wake in the night?
yes ☐ **no** ☐
As well as being exhausting, disturbed sleep is a sign of stress. See page 87 for advice on sleep patterns.

8 Do you regularly sleep less than seven hours a night?
yes ☐ **no** ☐
Sleep is essential for repairing the body and for its healthy functioning.

9 Do you exercise less than three times a week?
yes ☐ **no** ☐
Exercise has benefits for general health and hence for fertility (see pages 88–89).

10 Do you work long hours (more than 50 hours per week)?
yes ☐ **no** ☐
You should look at the reasons why you are working such long hours and find ways of improving the situation (see page 91).

11 Do you regularly work in the evenings or at the weekends?

yes ☐   **no** ☐

Working in the evenings is not conducive to a good night's sleep. Weekend working does not allow your brain to switch off and refresh itself in time for a new working week.

12 Do you worry about your finances?

yes ☐   **no** ☐

Financial worries put a strain on many couples. Aim to sort out your problems before they start to affect your health and your relationship (see page 91).

13 Do you dread the start of the working week?

yes ☐   **no** ☐

Look for ways to relax in anticipation of the week ahead, and assess whether you can change your work situation so that it causes you less anxiety.

14 Do you have little time to see friends and family?

yes ☐   **no** ☐

Spending time with those who are closest to you is mood-boosting, enjoyable, and relaxing, and helps to lower stress levels (see page 92).

15 Do you find it difficult to fit holidays into your work schedule?

yes ☐   **no** ☐

Holidays are essential if you need to wind down and reduce stress levels, and can be the best time to conceive (see page 93).

16 Do you find it difficult to switch off your mobile phone and be out of contact for a while?

yes ☐   **no** ☐

Learn to switch off from the outside world and to focus just on yourself and your partner.

your**score**

0–4 You have a reasonably balanced lifestyle, although you may have one or more areas of your life that need addressing. Make sure they are not affecting your overall health and chances of conceiving.

5–8 Your lifestyle is probably affecting your health and your fertility, even though it may not be apparent to you at the moment. Examine the different areas of your life that are problematic and re-read the advice on how to make the necessary changes in order to boost your fertility.

9–12 With only a few areas of your life actually in balance it's time to take stock and decide what is most important now that you are trying to start a family. The sooner you start to make improvements, the quicker the effects will be.

13–16 Your health and fertility are almost certainly affected already by your lifestyle. It is never too late to change and, with determination and planning, you can improve both immeasurably. Read through Steps 5, 6, and 7 carefully to find the quickest and most effective ways of transforming your lifestyle.

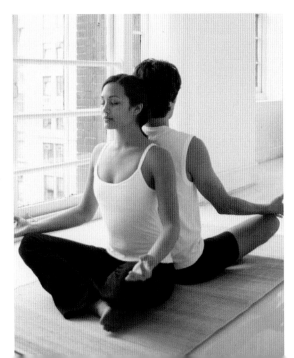

Nutrition is key when it comes to **being proactive** about your health – **take control** of what you eat and reap the **rewards**

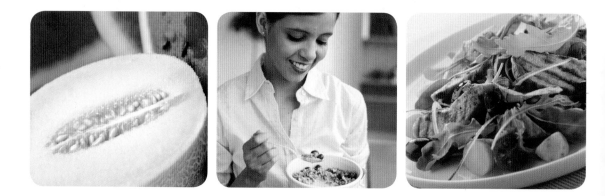

step**six**
eating to conceive

Your questions answered on:

step six: **eating to conceive**

Nutrition is a **key building block** of fertility. By giving careful consideration to what you eat and making changes where necessary, you will boost your chances of getting pregnant. **Make changes gradually**, focusing on one area at a time. In this way, you will be able to **get on with your life** without feeling under too much pressure

Q Is there a perfect diet to help couples boost their fertility?

When women start trying for a baby, and especially when they are having difficulty conceiving, they can easily become obsessed with what they eat. In no time at all, they start going on all sorts of unhealthy diets that needlessly exclude certain foods and encourage others, with no hard evidence that this approach will help them to conceive. These women either become confused or fixated about what they should and shouldn't eat. In addition, their diet can become bland and boring, and this can start to affect their mood, their socializing, and the pleasure they derive from food itself.

Food nourishes us on many different levels: it is not just sustenance. It feeds our senses and our emotions. The smell, sight, touch, and taste of food excites and satisfies us, and depriving yourself of this can make you feel low, frustrated, angry even, and can raise your levels of stress hormones. And none of these emotions is conducive to good health or to maximizing fertility.

I don't believe that the ultimate ideal balanced diet exists. I believe instead that people have good days and bad days, good weeks and bad weeks, and that the aim is to have a healthy diet that also leaves plenty of room for getting enjoyment from food. A lot of the

work I do with couples' dietary and lifestyle habits involves breaking vicious cycles and getting moderation back into their lives. The fundamental key is learning, or re-learning, to eat sensibly.

None of the changes you need to make can be done overnight, but with small, manageable moves in the right direction, much can be achieved to reach a sensible eating plan that will stay with you for good.

Q What do I need to be aware of to make sure my diet is healthy?

There are several things I advise clients to do when they are trying to improve their diet:

■ Make sure you eat things as close to their natural food state as possible. I don't believe in eating processed foods, foods containing refined sugars, or foods that are labelled "low-fat" or "no-fat" as these usually contain all sorts of added substances to make them more palatable.

■ Eat foods that are in season and fresh. Ideally, shop every couple of days rather than doing one big weekly supermarket shop that results in vegetables losing their freshness and a high proportion of their vitamins and minerals. You don't have to eat organic foods. In fact, it's better to make sure the meat you eat is free range rather than organic as it will have more taste. (You can have a battery chicken that is reared organically!)

■ Eat a wide variety of foods, and make sure they include lots of different colours. These will supply you with a wide range of vitamins and minerals.

■ If you have any dietary restrictions – if you are wheat-intolerant, for example – make sure you see a doctor or qualified nutritionist who can advise you about getting all the nutrients you need. Do not attempt to self-medicate.

Zita's **tip**

Rather than focusing on specific foods, aim for a **sensible overall healthy eating plan.**

Do not eliminate foods from your diet unless you are told to do so by a qualified doctor or nutritionist.

■ Have three meals a day: breakfast, lunch, and dinner. You can have a mid-morning and mid-afternoon snack, such as fresh or dried fruit, oatcakes, or mixed unsalted nuts and seeds, but avoid grazing on snacks such as crisps and biscuits throughout the day.

■ Drink plenty of water: many people don't drink enough water and often feel tired simply because they are mildly dehydrated. Adults should drink 2 litres (just over four pints) of water a day. Bear in mind that coffee and tea (apart from herbal and fruit teas) do not count as they have a diuretic effect and so rob your body of water.

Q Do I have to be at my ideal weight to get pregnant?

Not really. For the majority of women, their fertility is not affected by weighing a few kilos more than they would ideally like to. If this is the case for you, don't become obsessed about shedding a little excess fat.

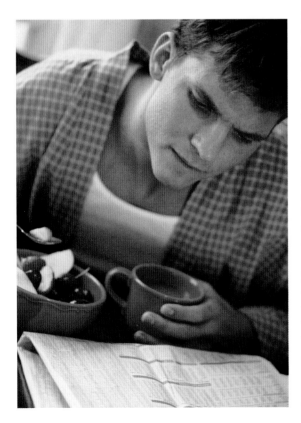

It is likely to make you miserable and will not improve your long-term chances of conceiving. Relax and simply try to adopt a healthy but enjoyable and achievable diet as soon as possible by following the guidelines set out in this step.

However, if your BMI is above 25 (see page 13), you could find your weight is impacting on your chances of getting pregnant. In this case, you need to seek professional help – rather than going on some unproven diet that is possibly harmful to your health and to your aim of getting pregnant – in order to rectify the situation before it becomes a potential problem. A good nutritionist will advise you on how to change your diet to achieve a healthy weight. This may take a few months, but for many women, even those whose BMI is significantly over 25, it can take a relatively short amount of time for their hormones to rebalance themselves, for their general health to improve and their fertility to be restored.

Q My BMI is low yet I am having trouble putting on weight. What can I do?

The ideal BMI is between 20 and 25. It is important to have a certain amount of body fat as reproductive hormones depend on fat for their production and metabolism. Insufficient fat may mean you are at a risk of producing too little oestrogen, and it can also cause a woman's eggs to develop poorly.

The key to healthy weight gain in preparation for pregnancy is to eat both calorie- and nutrient-rich foods – not to start filling up on nutrient-poor junk foods in order to put on weight. Eat three meals a day and include a mid-morning and a mid-afternoon snack, and one in the evening if necessary. It is important to include plenty of complex carbohydrates (see page 102) and some good-quality protein with each meal.

Avoid fizzy drinks, juices, tea, and coffee, which can fill you up. Include good-quality oils and fats, such as olive oil, avocados, all natural nuts and seeds, full-fat organic yogurt, and hummus. It is also essential to make sure that you are digesting your foods properly to be certain that all the important nutrients are absorbed – seek medical advice if you have problems with your digestion.

Both you and your partner need to be eating at least five varieties of fruit and vegetables a day to help keep you fit and healthy.

find out more: **a healthy diet**

Eating a healthy diet is easy as long as you **include a range of foods** chosen from each of the important food groups: carbohydrates, protein, fats, and fibre.

Opinions differ on the exact proportions between the groups but it is accepted that starchy carbohydrates such as bread, pasta, and potatoes should form the basis of your daily food intake. Carbohydrates are broken down in the body and turned into glucose, which supplies energy to all body cells. There are, however, some important distinctions between different types of carbohydrates (see page 102).

Fibre is essential for maintaining a good digestive system, for the slow, steady absorption of carbohydrates, and therefore for balancing blood sugar levels. Fresh fruit and vegetables are the best sources of fibre, as are unrefined carbohydrates such as wholegrain bread. Too much fibre, however, may lead to digestive problems and poor absorption of vital nutrients.

food group **percentages**

As a general rule, your diet should contain:

- 55 per cent complex carbohydrate
- 30 per cent fat
- 15 per cent protein (this is inclusive of at least five portions of fruit and vegetables a day to ensure enough fibre).
- You should also drink at least 2 litres (4 pints) of fluids a day (preferably water).

essential protein

The body's building blocks are proteins. These are large molecules made up of amino acids, which are necessary for cell growth and repair. There are 20 amino acids, of which eight are "essential" because our bodies cannot make them naturally, so we have to obtain them from food sources. Animal protein contains all these amino acids, as do soya products. Vegetable sources do not contain them all, so if you are on a vegan diet you need to ensure you are getting these by taking a vitamin

and mineral supplement or by combining pulses, nuts, and seeds with complex carbohydrates. Quinoa and avocado are complete proteins.

Women's protein requirements are lower than men's but they still need their daily diet to contain about 15 per cent of protein as it is an essential nutrient for muscle, tissue, and bone health, for helping to fight infection, for producing and balancing hormones, and for producing healthy eggs and sperm. Good sources of protein are chicken, fish, low-fat yogurt, cottage cheese, baked beans, kidney beans, tofu, and avocados.

One of the important amino acids for women is tryptophan, which helps in the production of the "feel-good" chemical serotonin, which is vital for regulating blood sugar and hormone levels (see pages 65 and 78). Women tend to be lower in serotonin than men, and so need to consume foods that will raise their levels. Foods rich in tryptophan include eggs, milk, and wholegrains. Serotonin is produced in larger quantities in the morning, which is why it is particularly important for women to eat breakfast.

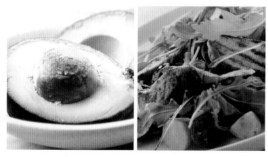

Avocado and chicken are good sources of protein.

the fat story

Women are brainwashed into thinking fats are bad but it all depends on what sort you eat and how much. Fat is needed to build cell walls, help the absorption of vitamins and nutrients and balance hormone and blood sugar levels.

Saturated and unsaturated fats Saturation refers to the number of hydrogen atoms attached to the fat molecule. When a fat molecule contains the maximum number of hydrogen atoms, it is "saturated". It is sometimes called a "hard" fat because it stays hard at room temperature. Saturated fats come from animal sources and are the least healthy and so should be eaten in moderation. If one pair of hydrogen atoms is missing, the molecule is said to be

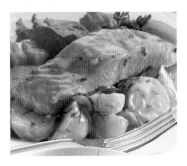

Oily fish such as mackerel, salmon, herrings, and sardines are the best dietary sources of omega-3.

monounsaturated – these fats are usually plant-based in origin. Olive oil is an example of a monounsaturated fat. If more than one pair of hydrogen atoms is missing, the fat is polyunsaturated – cooking oils for example. Both mono- and polyunsaturated fats are "healthy" fats.

Essential fatty acids Omega-3, omega-6, and omega-9 are unsaturated fats, essential for the production of prostaglandins, which are key to maintaining correct hormonal secretion and balance for both men and women. These essential fatty acids are also important for the production of serotonin. Olive oil, for example, contains omega-6 and omega-9 oils. Omega-3 oil, found in oily fish, walnuts, pumpkins, and sesame seeds, is particularly important for healthy cell metabolism, brain function, healthy sperm production and heart health.

Hydrogenated fats and transfats When a hydrogen atom is added to an unsaturated vegetable fat, the molecule is then referred to as "hydrogenated" and the fat becomes a "transfat". These unnatural fats, found in many junk foods, biscuits, and cakes, are difficult for the body to digest and metabolize, and carry known health risks.

in praise of dairy

Milk has several clear-cut nutritional benefits. It is a major source of calcium, particularly in its semi-skimmed or skimmed versions (because these contain a lower percentage of fat). Calcium is essential for healthy bones and muscles, as well as for the good functioning of nerve impulses.

There are other dietary sources of calcium, including green vegetables, seeds, and certain breads, but calcium from milk is more easily absorbed by the body. You would have to eat 16 portions of spinach, for example, to get as much calcium as you get from one 240ml (8fl oz) glass of milk. Milk is also an excellent source of the essential B group of vitamins and of protein. Drink skimmed or semi-skimmed milk to reduce the quantity of saturated fat.

Live yogurt is recommended in the diet as it is easily digestible. Some cheese in the diet is also fine, although you should avoid high-fat cheeses and always try to buy organic dairy produce.

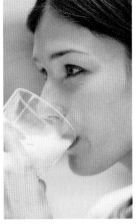

Milk provides several essential nutrients – don't limit your intake when trying to get pregnant.

0.5%
fat content in **skimmed milk**

The lower the fat content, the more calcium and protein in the milk. Vitamin D, which is a fat-soluble vitamin, helps with the absorption of calcium from milk.

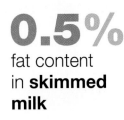

Q I try to avoid carbohydrates but is a carb-free or low-carb diet a bad idea?

If you avoid carbohydrates you may start to feel low, depressed, or lethargic as a result of low serotonin levels. Serotonin, as well as other neurotransmitters (chemicals that transmit messages from one nerve cell to another), such as endorphins and encephalins, are present throughout the body, especially in the brain, digestive tract, and uterus. Along with oestrogen, they help the lining of the uterus to develop and prepare it for an implanting embryo.

Q What is the link between carbohydrates and adrenaline?

If your blood sugar level drops because your carbohydrate intake is restricted, adrenaline is secreted to counter this. Because adrenaline is a stress hormone it can lead to hormone disruption, which impacts on your fertility (see page 84). In addition, stress and adrenaline secretion use up valuable amounts of magnesium, zinc, and the B group of vitamins, all of which are essential for good health. The adrenal glands also need a constant supply of vitamin C and essential fatty acids, and the body's store of them gets depleted if too much adrenaline is produced.

Q Should I cut out sugary foods?

In order to break the cycle of dependence on sugary or high-energy foods, such as cake, pastry or chocolate, it is important to cut out – at least for a two-week period – all refined and simple sugars and to substitute them with complex carbohydrates (see below) and low GI foods (see facing page). At first, you may feel light-headed or dizzy, and you may get headaches, but persevere.

Make sure you eat three proper meals a day (never skip breakfast), and have some low GI snacks for mid-morning and mid-afternoon to help you to keep your blood sugar levels balanced. By the end of this time you will realize that some parts of your diet may not even have had to change much, simply substituting, for example, brown rice or wholegrain bread for white rice or white bread, and this will make it easier to make these alterations permanent. You will also notice that supposedly high-energy, high-sugar snacks were responsible for some big energy lows as well, and that you are now able to keep going for longer by switching to eating complex carbohydrates.

Only once you have rebalanced your blood sugar levels can you occasionally reintroduce some simple carbohydrates into your diet. But as the idea is to re-educate your palate, there is no point in slipping back into previous bad habits.

Q What are **"good"** and **"bad"** carbohydrates?

Understanding the difference between simple ("bad") and complex ("good") carbohydrates will help you make sure your diet contains sufficient quantities of the carbs your body needs for sustained energy production.

Simple carbohydrates are easily broken down, giving quick-release energy. They raise blood sugar and insulin levels fast, but this is followed by a drop in blood sugar, leading to a physical need for yet more sugar to reverse the unpleasant feelings this produces (dizziness, mood swings, lack of concentration, irritability). Simple carbs include all sugar and sweet foods, sugary drinks and alcohol, foods made from refined carbohydrates, and many processed foods. Refined carbohydrates (white bread, white flour, and white rice) have had the fibre removed and thus some of the beneficial nutrients.

Some fruit, such as bananas and watermelon, and some fruit juices and smoothies, also have a high sugar content and give an immediate energy boost.

Complex carbohydrates consist of sugar molecules linked together and these take longer to be broken down and carried in the bloodstream because they require a specific enzyme to do so. This means that the blood sugar level rises slowly and energy release is slow. Then levels drop gradually, avoiding the blood sugar slump that makes people crave more sugar.

Beans, pulses, and fruit such as apples, pears, peaches, and plums are good sources of complex carbohydrates, as are starchy foods such as brown rice, and wholegrain bread, which have retained their vitamins and minerals along with their fibre.

find out more: **the glycaemic index**

The glycaemic index (GI) is an index, on a scale of 1 to 100, based on how quickly a food is digested, metabolized, and then released into the bloodstream as glucose. It is a useful indicator of which foods are slow-releasing and will help to keep your blood sugar levels stable.

Low GI foods have the slowest release of energy and you should eat as many of these as possible. Medium GI foods can be eaten in moderation and high GI foods should be eaten the least frequently and ideally with protein or fats to slow their absorption.

The lists below are not exhaustive, but you can see that some fruit have a lower GI rating than some vegetables, so the information can be a helpful way to ensure that you avoid the yo-yo effect of high and low blood sugar levels. The foods at the end of the high GI list are refined and processed, or have added sweeteners, and should be avoided wherever possible.

how to keep the **GI low**

- Very ripe or overripe fruit has a high sugar content, so try to avoid eating fruit in this state.
- Potatoes that have been cooked then cooled have a lower GI content than just-cooked potatoes.

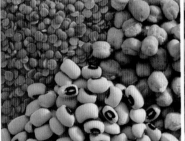

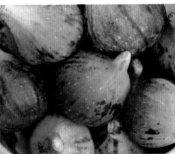

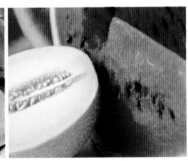

Low GI foods (40 and under)
Eat as many of these slow-releasing foods as you wish.

- Apples, plums, pears, peaches, cherries, apricots (fresh and dried), grapefruit
- All pulses: red lentils, kidney beans, baked beans, chick peas, cannelloni beans, pearl barley
- Green leafy vegetables, broccoli, leeks, cauliflower, green beans, mangetout
- Mushrooms, onions, avocados, courgettes, peppers
- Whole cereals, wholegrain or rye bread, barley, nuts, oat biscuits

Medium GI foods (41–60)
These are fine for you to eat in moderate amounts.

- Grapes, underripe bananas, mangoes, figs, kiwi fruit, sultanas
- Sweetcorn, peas, raw carrots, beetroot, boiled potatoes with skins, sweet potatoes, baked beans in tomato sauce
- Wholemeal noodles, popcorn, wholewheat pasta, brown basmati rice, wholemeal spaghetti
- Stoneground wholemeal bread, pitta bread
- Muesli (non toasted)
- Orange juice, grapefruit juice, unsweetened apple juice

High GI foods (over 60)
Eat those at the beginning of the list in moderation, preferably in conjunction with protein or fat as these slow down the absorption of carbohydrates.

- Ripe bananas, watermelon, raisins, pineapple, cantaloupe
- Baked potatoes, mashed potatoes, cooked carrots, parsnip, swede, squash, broad beans

Avoid the following:
- French fries
- Couscous
- Sugar, honey, chocolate, sweets, jam, sugared breakfast cereals, rice cakes
- White bread, rice, and pasta

Q Why are vitamins and minerals so important to fertility?

Vitamins and minerals are vital for your overall health and in particular for your fertility, but there seems to be an enormous amount of confusion among my clients regarding which ones they should be taking and in what doses. The chart below should help.

Vitamins and minerals provide you with the essential nutrients to allow your body to function to its maximum capacity; they help keep your hormones balanced; they provide energy; they help growth and repair cell damage; and their antioxidant qualities neutralize the harmful effects of free radicals.

Q What are free radicals?

Free radicals are the "loose", unstable molecules in cells that try to stabilize themselves by oxidizing molecules around them, thereby causing "rust-like" damage. Free radicals are implicated in diseases such as cancer and heart disorders. They occur naturally, and are part of the ageing process, but environmental pollutants such as smoking, and alcohol and bad diet increase the amount of free radical damage to your body. Furthermore, free radicals damage sperm and egg production, which is another reason why smoking and alcohol reduce women's fertile years and lower men's sperm counts. More and more research is being done into the role that free radicals play in fertility and pregnancy.

Q Which are the key **vitamins** and **minerals**?

The five main vitamins are A, B, C, D, and E and, apart from vitamin D, can only be obtained from the food we eat. In addition to the list below, there are many other minerals, including magnesium, manganese, potassium, co-enzyme Q_{10}, and calcium, which contribute to health and fertility.

I truly believe that the best way to ensure that you are not deficient in any vitamin or mineral is to eat a diet that is as varied and healthy as possible. Antioxidants, for example, work best when they interact with other vitamins and minerals and that is best achieved by a diverse, nutritious diet.

the main minerals and vitamins

mineral or vitamin	found in	good for
Vitamin A	Egg yolk, oily fish, butter, orange fruit and vegetables (peaches, apricots, carrots, mangoes); vegetable products contain high doses of vitamin A in the betacarotene form (as do pre-pregnancy vitamin supplements) and these are safe to eat.	Healthy skin, eyes, bones; production of male and female sex hormones; helping to fight infection; antioxidant properties. **Warning:** high doses of vitamin A in a form called retinol can cause fetal abnormalities; avoid liver and liver products which contain this form of vitamin A. Vitamin A is no longer included in pre-conception products.
Vitamin B$_1$ (thiamine)	Potatoes, wholegrains, pulses, brown rice.	Converting carbs and fats into energy (B vitamins work together and should be taken as a complex).
Vitamin B$_6$	Bananas, avocados, lean meat, milk products, eggs, seeds, lentils, wholegrains.	Balance of female sex hormones (vitamin B$_6$ deficiency causes the ovaries to stop producing progesterone, leading to oestrogen dominance).

Q Should I be taking a vitamin and mineral supplement?

If you are eating a healthy, balanced diet and are not smoking, drinking, or consuming too much caffeine (see page 108), then you probably do not need to be taking any supplements, other than folic acid. However, as an "insurance policy" I often advise that women could take a specific pre-pregnancy multivitamin supplement and men a general supplement. This will ensure that they are not deficient in any vitamin or mineral and that they are taking them at safe doses too. Sometimes when people start to self-medicate and take a supplement for one or more vitamins or minerals, they end up taking needlessly

large doses. Ironically, these large doses can interact with other substances in the body and be harmful to health and fertility. So, you should never self-medicate with individual supplements of specific vitamins and minerals. Consult a nutritional therapist (who is trained to know which supplements can safely be added to the diet) or a pharmacist if you are in doubt about what you intend to take. All women planning a pregnancy should be taking 400mcg of folic acid for at least 12 weeks before conception and for the first 12 weeks of pregnancy, as this has been proven to reduce the risk of having a baby with a neural tube defect such as spina bifida. Check that your pre-pregnancy multivitamin contains the recommended amount of folic acid. Women with some medical disorders,

mineral or vitamin	found in	good for
Vitamin B_{12}	Animal protein (meat, fish, and dairy foods).	Maintaining sperm count; helping to form cell DNA and RNA (ribonucleic acid, which allows cells to duplicate); iron absorption; ripening eggs prior to ovulation.
Vitamin C	Fruit and vegetables, especially citrus fruit, berries, kiwi fruit, kale, broccoli, spinach, cabbage.	Antioxidant properties; iron absorption; supporting immune system; promoting healthy, motile sperm; protecting ovarian health. **Warning:** women should not take more than 1,000mg vitamin C a day because large doses may dry up cervical secretions.
Vitamin D	Oily fish, butter, egg yolks; also from exposure to daylight.	Strong, healthy bones and teeth; absorption of calcium.
Vitamin E	Wholegrains, nuts, seeds, eggs.	Antioxidant properties; healthy skin, nerves, muscles, red blood cells; male and female fertility.
Iron	Lean meat, broccoli, spinach, dried apricots, prunes, sardines, oatmeal, eggs.	Maintaining levels of red blood cells and keeping blood oxygenated; energy; female fertility. (Iron from animal sources is absorbed in greater quantities than iron from vegetables – vitamin C-rich foods help absorption).
Zinc	Lean meat, fish, eggs, pumpkin and sunflower seeds, peas, rye, oats, almonds.	Sperm and egg production; healthy cell division and immune system; sperm count and motility; healthy menstrual cycle.
Selenium	Brazil nuts, eggs, meat, fish, sunflower seeds, butter, oats.	Antioxidant properties; male and female fertility; healthy sperm; preventing chromosomal abnormalities.

Q What are the **top superfoods for** fertility?

No foods can be guaranteed to enhance your chances of conceiving. However, there are plenty of good things to eat that can have a positive impact on your health. Some foods are thought to reduce the risk of problems related to fertility in both women and men.

Sex and libido foods For centuries, certain foods have been associated with sexual desire and fertility, mainly because they are thought to resemble the shape of the sexual organs. These foods include pomegranates, avocados, bananas, figs, dates, asparagus, almonds, garlic, and oysters. Whether or not they work as aphrodisiacs, as is sometimes claimed, is open to debate. However, they are certainly rich in vital vitamins and minerals that are good for fertility.

Brain foods Eating foods containing the amino acids tryptophan and tyrosine may raise levels of the brain chemicals serotonin and dopamine. These chemicals play a role in the production of hormones that prepare the uterus to receive an embryo. Tryptophan is found in parsley, papaya, dates, bananas, celery, spirulina, carrots, dried apricots, sweet potatoes, sunflower seeds, and almonds. For foods supplying tyrosine, try lean meats turkey, fish – such as cod, sea bass, and sardines – crab, kidney or mung beans, and oats.

Foods to protect sperm and eggs Sperm cells and egg cells are highly susceptible to damage by free radicals. Eating foods that are rich in flavanoids helps to protect them. Flavanoids are a group of plant pigments that give colour to a whole range of fruits and have potent antioxidant activity, which helps to neutralize the damage caused by free radicals. Blueberries, raspberries, cherries, grapes, oranges, peaches, plums, and tomatoes are all good sources of flavanoids.

Sperm-boosting foods Lack of certain nutrients can affect a man's production of sperm. Two of the most important dietary elements for improving numbers and quality of sperm are zinc and vitamin C. Good sources of zinc include brazil nuts, eggs, fish, and seeds and grains. Foods rich in vitamin C include green leafy vegetables, kiwi fruit, and tomatoes.

Foods for healthy secretions The secretions a woman produces each month are alkaline, as is the environment in which sperm are transported. A fertility diet should be rich in high-alkaline foods, which include many fruits and vegetables. Try asparagus, bamboo shoots, broccoli, carrots, cabbage, celery, cucumbers, leeks, onions, potatoes, apples, avocados, cherries, mangoes, olives, and peaches.

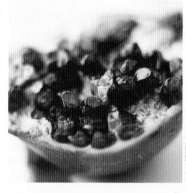

Symbol of fertility in many ancient cultures, the pomegranate contains antioxidants and several vitamins, and is rich in iron.

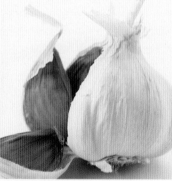

Garlic is packed with vitamins A, B, and C and is a good source of health-boosting minerals such as zinc and potassium.

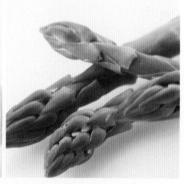

Asparagus provides folates, which guard against birth defects, so this is an excellent food if you are planning a pregnancy.

such as epilepsy, may require a higher dose of folic acid – discuss this with your doctor.

Finally, if you are on any form of prescribed medication for a specific medical condition, always consult a doctor if you are thinking of taking any vitamin or mineral supplement, as these could interact negatively with the drugs you are taking.

Q I eat healthily but don't seem to feel the benefits – why is that?

Choosing the right food is important but the way you live your life has a direct bearing on how effective your diet is – excessive stress, for example, drains your body of vitamin C. Similarly, alcohol and caffeine (especially in coffee and tea) deplete the body's stores of many vitamins and minerals, including B vitamins, zinc, and calcium. Smoking depletes the body of vitamins C and E. If you generally feel low and rundown, your lifestyle could be neutralizing many of the benefits of eating healthily.

Q Which is better for me – acidic or alkaline food?

To achieve good health and enhance fertility it is essential to ensure that your body is in an alkaline rather than an acid state. Many of us eat far too many acidic foods, such as excessive amounts of animal protein, sugar, fat, alcohol, caffeine, and artifical chemicals, as well as refined carbohydrates. Indeed, weight loss diets based on high-protein foods (meat, fish, eggs, and dairy) are bad for women trying to become pregnant. These diets can deprive the body of minerals such as calcium, magnesium, and potassium, which are needed in large reserves to buffer the body against over-acidity. Drinking soft, carbonated drinks is not recommended as they contain phosphorus and are rather acidic. As a result, calcium can be leached from the bones in order to prevent over-acidity, which in turn leads to an increased risk of osteoporosis. It is therefore important to include in your diet plenty of alkaline-forming foods, such as fresh fruit and vegetables, certain nuts, seeds and grains, and to drink plenty of water.

Q Which **additives** should be avoided?

It is not possible to eliminate all additives from the food you eat, but you should aim to cut them out wherever possible. Always look at food labels: as a basic rule, the fewer the number of ingredients listed the purer the food.

Salt This is the number one food additive that everyone should avoid consuming to excess. A diet that is high in salt can lead to high blood pressure and, because of the impact on health, this can affect fertility adversely, and male fertility in particular (see page 52).

Cut down on high-salt foods, including items such as crisps and salted nuts, and also beware of the hidden sources of salt, namely in convenience and take-away foods, and in apparently harmless foods such as bread and cereals, many of which contain surprisingly high amounts. When cooking, avoid adding salt to the food. In no time at all you can re-educate your palate to get used to a less salty taste of all the foods that you consume.

Aspartame and other artificial sweeteners
These are found in sweet diet foods and drinks. Some studies suggest a link between aspartame and depression, weight gain, and possibly even infertility and miscarriage, so this additive is best avoided when trying to conceive.

Acrylamide This is produced when certain starchy foods, notably potatoes, are fried at high temperature, as is the case with chips and crisps. It has been shown to reduce fertility in rats and to be carcinogenic for animals, so avoid, or at least cut down on, these foods.

Monosodium glutamate (MSG) and certain preservatives, artificial colourings, and flavourings These are used to enhance the flavour and look of food, or to replace natural ingredients. Although many additives and preservatives are deemed "safe", it may be that a combination can have adverse effects within the body. If a food label has a long list of substances you can't identify, avoid it.

Q What effect does caffeine have on metabolism?

Caffeine is a stimulant that enters the bloodstream approximately 15 minutes after consumption. It causes the pituitary gland to instruct the adrenal glands to secrete adrenaline and, as a result, caffeine slightly increases both blood pressure and heart rate. It is also a diuretic, which means it stimulates urination and depletes the body of fluid. The caffeine content of a cup of coffee or tea varies considerably, depending on the serving size, the method of preparation, and even the type of coffee bean or tea leaves used. Chocolate (especially milk chocolate) and cocoa also contain caffeine, although at low levels. About one hour after consumption, the effects of the caffeine have ceased, your raised blood sugar levels (caused by adrenaline) have dropped again and you start to crave another shot of stimulant. You may also feel a bit weary due to the diuretic, or draining, effect, which compounds the feeling of needing another dose of caffeine.

Q What effect does caffeine have on fertility and in pregnancy?

Some studies have found a link between high levels of caffeine consumption in women and a delay in conceiving. Those who consumed more than 300mg of caffeine per day – the equivalent of two cups of fresh coffee (see below) – were more likely to have a delay in conceiving. It is still unclear whether it is safe to consume caffeine before and during pregnancy and, if so, in what quantities. As a precaution, you should aim to cut down on caffeine as much as possible while you are trying to get pregnant.

There is also some evidence to suggest that drinking large amounts of caffeine during pregnancy may increase the risk of miscarriage.

Q How should I go about reducing my caffeine intake?

People who are regular consumers of caffeine, especially those who drink a lot of coffee every day, may suffer side effects when they stop. These can include extreme tiredness, nausea, headaches, dizziness, trembling hands, and mood swings. To avoid this, or at least to minimize the withdrawal symptoms, I would advise you to cut down gradually, by two cups a week for example, until you have eliminated caffeine altogether.

Q How can I monitor what I eat and drink?

Now that you know more about what makes up a healthy diet, it is a good idea to keep a food diary to identify trends and tendencies in what you eat. If you note down everything you eat and drink over a period of seven days, you will get a clearer idea of whether you are eating healthily or whether you need to make some adjustments to your diet.

Write down everything you eat and drink (and that includes alcohol!), even if you have just had a mouthful or a sip. For example, you might have dipped into a bowl of crisps in the pub and, without realizing, raised your intake of salt and saturated fats that day, or you might have half drunk several cups of coffee or cans of fizzy drink at work and ended up consuming rather more caffeine than you imagined.

Looking at the balance of healthy versus unhealthy foods, does the former significantly outweigh the latter? Are you eating five or more portions of fruit and vegetables a day? Are you eating significantly more lean meat than fatty meat? How many times a week do you eat convenience or take-away foods? Do the results come as a surprise to you?

Nobody is an angel when it comes to food, but you probably know by looking at the results of your food diary where your diet could improve. Concentrate on making the changes you need to boost your overall health and your chances of conceiving.

how much caffeine?

drink	caffeine
240ml (8oz) cup of brewed coffee	150mg
240ml (8oz) cup of instant coffee	100mg
240ml (8oz) cup of tea	60 to 90mg
355ml (12oz) can of caffeinated fizzy drink	35 to 40mg
28g (1oz) of dark chocolate	20mg

Q What is the difference between food allergy and food intolerance?

A food allergy develops when the body reacts to a normally harmless substance, mistaking it for a dangerous one. The immune system kicks in, producing antibodies that trigger the release of histamine. Fortunately, it is still quite rare to be truly allergic to a specific food or food group and people who do have such an allergy are never left in any doubt: within minutes of ingesting the food, their body's immune system reacts violently and produces symptoms such as an itchy rash, hives, swelling, even difficulty breathing and/or a massive drop in blood pressure. In severe cases, the reaction can prove fatal. The most common foods that cause allergies are peanuts, other types of nuts, fish, shellfish, and eggs.

In addition to food allergies, a growing number of people are becoming intolerant to certain foods, in particular wheat and dairy products, although the true numbers are disputed, even by doctors who work solely in this field. Many causes are suggested, including environmental pollutants, chemicals in the foods themselves, our immune system, and our increasingly antiseptic environment. A food intolerance would typically produce one or several delayed symptoms, ranging from asthma, eczema, migraines, and headaches to tiredness and digestive disorders. If you suspect you may have symptoms of a food intolerance, you should either ask your GP to refer you to a specialist allergy clinic at your local hospital, or make an appointment to see a qualified dietician who will arrange for you to have some tests.

Q Does a food allergy or intolerance have an impact on fertility?

Food intolerance or allergy can affect the way the body absorbs nutrients, so you may be losing out on some of the vitamins and minerals that assist fertility. If you are sure that you are affected, it is important to avoid the foods that may be causing problems. If you suspect an intolerance, make sure you are properly tested before you eliminate anything from your diet. Don't just cut food groups out of your diet without finding the specific culprit and including appropriate alternatives.

Q What are the common **food intolerances**?

There is hardly a food on earth that does not cause intolerance in somebody. Foods as diverse as citrus fruit and chocolates are often cited, but the two most common foods that are suspected of producing food intolerances are those containing milk (and associated dairy products) and gluten.

Cow's milk A few people are indeed intolerant of cow's milk, but the vast majority of people are able to consume it safely. Human beings are born with the enzyme needed to digest the lactose present in human milk and other mammal milk. If our diet does not include milk after weaning (as is the case with many Asian diets), the body tells itself that the enzyme, produced in the gut, is no longer required. It stops being produced and intolerance to dairy produce then develops. Milk intolerance, if it does develop and if it is severe, usually becomes apparent early in life. Substituting goat's milk for cow's milk makes no difference because the same allergens are present in goat's milk. Soya milk is increasingly used as a dairy alternative but, again, you should be aware that intolerance and even allergy to soya products is on the increase in the Western world, and usually begins once soya becomes a frequently consumed food, so it may not be a suitable long-term alternative.

Gluten This is a protein contained in wheat, rye, barley, and oats, although the latter contain low quantities. People who suffer symptoms such as diarrhoea, bloating, abdominal pain, and general lethargy may suspect they are intolerant of gluten. However, it is essential that they consult a medically qualified expert in order to find out if this is the case. It will do more harm to your overall health if you exclude wheat, rye, barley, and oats from your diet without firm evidence that you need to because you could be depriving your body of essential nutrients and impacting on your chances of conceiving.

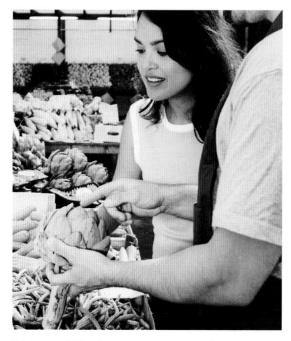

It is important that the fruit and vegetables you buy are as fresh as possible. If they are also organically grown, then even better.

Q Should all my food be organic?

Organic food is expensive and it is difficult to afford to eat exclusively organic. I always tell clients that the most important thing is to buy fresh. So, rather than doing one big weekly supermarket shop try to shop every couple of days to ensure freshness. If you are in a position to buy some organic food, the best products to choose are meat and dairy. Eat a wide variety of foods, particularly different coloured fruit and vegetables, rather than limit yourself to only one or two organic products. Make sure you always wash your fruit and vegetables thoroughly.

Q What are the effects of poor digestion on health and fertility?

I really believe that fertility and hormonal balance are influenced by the digestive system. Bad digestion leads to poor absorption of essential nutrients, as well as tiredness and lack of energy. Your immune system can become depleted as a result, and this can make you more prone to infections and illnesses. Indeed, there is an increased risk of developing a food intolerance or allergy when the immune

system is weakened, and if you are already intolerant or allergic to a particular food you may react more strongly to it. Moreover, poor diet can affect your hormonal secretion and therefore your chances of conceiving.

Q What are the causes of bad digestion?

Symptoms of poor digestion include constipation, bloating, diarrhoea, flatulence, and heartburn. The causes can be diverse but can either be the result of your lifestyle, a medical condition, or a food intolerance.

First, you should assess your lifestyle and ask yourself certain key questions:
- Do you eat late at night?
- Do you eat large amounts in the evening?
- Do you eat in a hurry or "on the go"?
- Is your diet too rich in fatty foods?
- Do you drink too much alcohol?
- Are you under a lot of stress?
- Do you regularly eat processed or junk food?
- Do you eat fewer than three portions of fruit or vegetables per day?

If you have answered "yes" to any of these questions, your lifestyle may be a key factor. Read Step 5 to see how you can make lifestyle changes that will improve your digestion, and make sure you improve your diet as well so that it can benefit your health and ultimately your fertility.

If addressing these issues doesn't resolve your digestive problems, then you need to consult a doctor in order to rule out any underlying medical cause. Similarly, if you think the problem could lie with a food intolerance, you should seek a proper medical opinion to try and find out which food or foods could be responsible.

Q Why do I find it so difficult to be consistent about what I eat?

Women's diets, much more than men's, are affected by their moods and energy levels. When women are tired, under stress, anxious, or upset, they often crave sugary and/or starchy foods, and start to eat unhealthily. But the time when women's dietary habits really fluctuate the most is usually just before their periods start. It is estimated that 40 per cent of women experience pre-menstrual syndrome (PMS) and it appears that hormones, notably progesterone, oestrogen, and testosterone, as well as the chemical serotonin, provoke changes in the brain that make women crave carbohydrates (see page 102). The desire for sweet foods is increased because these are a quick and easy way to raise the levels of serotonin and mood-enhancing endorphins but the effects are very short term (see page 106).

Q How can I avoid food cravings?

It is fine to eat carbohydrates to satisfy food cravings, just avoid eating simple or refined carbs that will make your blood sugar levels yo-yo and will lead to further cravings, weight gain, and hormonal imbalance. Instead, try eating complex carbs with, if possible, some protein to slow down the absorption, keep the blood sugar level stable and reduce further cravings. For example, try eating some nuts or cheese (both are proteins) with fruit, or eat some dried apricots with a glass of milk.

■ Another good way of cutting down on food cravings caused by mood swings or hormonal changes is to eat little and often, to keep your blood sugar at an even level throughout the day and avoid it getting too low.

■ Keep to a regular schedule and never skip a meal.
■ Keep up your levels of calcium and magnesium by eating foods such as dairy products (for calcium), pulses (for magnesium), and green leafy vegetables (for both), as these have been reported to cut symptoms of PMS by 40 to 50 per cent.
■ Make sure you drink plenty of water and exercise, even moderately, at least three times a week (see page 90).
■ Try to avoid situations that trigger food cravings. If you always feel like sugar on your way home from work, prepare a tempting, healthy snack before you set off, so that you don't give in to the chocolate bar impulse.

Q Why do women often have a difficult relationship with food?

Entire books have been written on the subject of our relationship with food, and women often have particular problems. Very few women are totally at ease with food, and as many as 30 per cent are on a diet

how to **improve your digestion**

There are several ways in which you can improve your digestion, and most of these involve making relatively simple changes to your eating habits.

■ Eat a proper breakfast. In traditional Chinese Medicine it is believed that 7am to 9am are the peak hours for the stomach to digest.
■ Complex carbohydrates, such as brown rice and beans and pulses, are best avoided in the middle of the day, as they can make you sleepy. If you do eat them – for example, if you regularly have a lunchtime sandwich – make sure you also eat plenty of lean protein as well to keep you going. Protein contains the amino acid tryptophan, which in turn helps with the production of serotonin (see page 100). Carbohydrates, on the other hand, trigger the production of serotonin, a "feel-good" chemical that is also important for the lining of the uterus.
■ Give yourself at least two hours, and preferably four, to digest your evening meal. Do not eat too much at dinner (or at any other meal, for that matter). The evening is the hardest time to digest

food, as that is when the body is slowing down metabolically, in readiness for sleep.
■ The stomach digests food 50 per cent more slowly at night than during the day, so avoid going to bed on a full stomach.
■ Avoid eating hard-to-digest raw foods in the evening. Eat raw fruit earlier in the day.
■ Avoid eating in a hurry or on the go. I'm always amazed by the amount of food – including lunch – that gets eaten while people are moving about. Again, this is not conducive to good digestion.
■ Eat when you are hungry and stop eating when you have had enough. Don't feel you always have to finish what is on your plate. You could end up feeling completely bloated by the end of the meal.
■ Chew slowly! Take your time eating. Part of the digestion process begins in the mouth with the various enzymes present in saliva. If you swallow food too fast, the process has not had a chance to get going properly. Also, by chewing properly and taking longer to eat, you will feel fuller more quickly, and you will eat less as a result.

at any one time. However, if you are planning to get pregnant it is important to avoid dieting – unless you need to lose weight in order to improve your fertility (see pages 13 and 99) – and to make healthy eating your number one priority.

Many women have an emotional relationship with food: they overeat or eat the wrong foods when they're depressed, anxious, under stress, or when they are affected by hormonal imbalances, especially when these are caused by premenstrual syndrome (PMS).

If you find that your diet is regularly affected by your fluctuating moods, you most likely have issues with food and will need to look at and try to understand the emotional reasons why you have bad dietary habits. This can take time and may need specialist help, but your health and your fertility will both benefit from trying to develop a better approach to food.

Q Can eating disorders affect fertility?

Some women have issues with food that go beyond regular dieting. These eating disorders – namely anorexia and bulimia – are increasingly common and their effects are potentially catastrophic for a woman's fertility. It is not within the scope of this book to advise women on how to tackle such serious disorders, as these usually stem from deep-seated psychological problems. If you suffer from an eating disorder, you will need to seek professional help because you may find it difficult to get pregnant, as your hormonal balance may be affected. If your body weight and body fat percentage are very low you may have ceased to have periods completely or you may have irregular periods and this could reduce your chances of conception. If you do conceive while seriously underweight, your body

case**study**

Amanda and David have been trying for a baby for 18 months. Amanda has suffered from anorexia in the past and her current BMI is just 17.

Amanda I have always had food issues, going right back to my teens, and at one stage it really got out of hand and my parents had to seek professional help for me. Now I'm trying to get pregnant I realize the impact all this has had on my body. I am still very controlled about what I eat and I am a bit obsessive about exercise – I go running five or six times a week. I do realize that if I want to get pregnant I need to make changes on every level, but I am really nervous about putting on weight during pregnancy, even though I know I have to.

I find it very disheartening when family and friends tell me I'll never get pregnant because I am too thin and this sets off my cycle again. David also gets frustrated with my eating habits, especially when we go out to dinner, and this can cause a lot of tension.

When I began to think I would never get pregnant, we both went to an appointment at the Zita West Clinic and I am now learning to understand the link between body fat and fertility, which I hadn't appreciated before. My periods have always been irregular but I thought that the fact that I was having them at all meant I was ovulating and

could conceive. I now realise that this isn't necessarily the case.

I was very apprehensive about undertaking the nutritional programme – I often feel more obsessive when people tell me what I can and can't eat. But it was made easier by having simple steps to follow and building in different aspects on a week-by-week basis. I have also cut down on my running and am receiving counselling to help address my food issues.

Seeing Zita helps David, too. He is working hard to understand my problems and to be supportive, and also appreciates the effort I am making to change.

Now, my BMI is rising, my periods have become more regular and I feel on a much more even keel. I am increasingly optimistic about my chances of getting pregnant, although it hasn't happened yet.

There are always underlying emotional issues surrounding eating disorders and these need to be addressed on all levels if fertility is to be improved.

could be depleted in several key nutrients and this could impact on your baby's health.

I see and help a lot of women with eating disorders who do go on to conceive, but usually they need a lot of support and have to make significant lifestyle changes to achieve their much-wanted pregnancy.

Q When will the changes I have made to my diet start to make a difference?

Whatever dietary changes you have or have not made, my aim in the course of this step has been to show you that it is perfectly possible to eat a diet that is not only healthy but also varied and enjoyable. And that by doing so, you will be doing all you can to improve your fertility.

When you make changes, don't try to do everything at once. Make them gradually and they will be easier to sustain. Within three to four months you should start to notice an improvement in your fertility. For general health, you can often notice an improvement in as little as a couple of weeks. Hopefully, too, the changes you have made to your diet are permanent, and this will also benefit your long-term health.

Q What is the best way to shop for a healthy diet?

You can only eat healthily if you have the ingredients to do so in the first place. Many people are bored by the notion of the weekly shop, and find themselves buying more or less the same things week in, week out. It is easy to get into a rut as far as your diet is concerned. Yet, boredom is one of the enemies of healthy eating, as is poor planning.

Ideally, you should give some thought to what you plan to eat, make a list, then aim to shop a little and often in order to maintain maximum freshness of the food you buy. Decide to try out one new recipe each week, for example, and shop accordingly: this will maintain your interest in food and motivate you to keep eating healthily.

If you have a local butcher, buy your meat there so you can get used to the different cuts. This will enable you to discover which ones are lean and will also lead to you cooking a wider range of dishes than if you bought your meat from a supermarket. Similarly, fishmongers will provide you with a far bigger choice of interesting fish and shellfish than even the best-stocked supermarkets, and they will be happy to offer advice on different ways to cook it.

When it comes to fruit and vegetables, you should aim for a variety of of colours and textures instead of always buying the same ones, so that you benefit from the maximum range of vitamins and minerals. Indeed, one of the keys to healthy eating is to eat as varied a diet as possible. In this way, you will maximize your chances of obtaining all your essential nutrients from food alone.

Finally, avoid shopping on an empty stomach or when you are tired, as this encourages you to buy unhealthy foods and to start snacking on them before you get home.

your new **golden rules**

By now, you should have adopted a healthier diet and may be surprised by how much you are enjoying your food and looking forward to mealtimes. Certain aspects of your food shopping and eating are likely to have changed too:

- You are shopping little and often, to maximize freshness of food.
- You are eating produce that is in season.
- You have cut out processed and convenience foods.
- You are eating five portions of fresh fruit or vegetables a day.
- The carbohydrates you are eating are complex and unrefined.
- You eat red meat no more than twice a week.
- You avoid fatty meat such as lamb and have switched to lean cuts of beef. Game such as venison is low in fat, as is poultry.
- You eat nuts, seeds, and dried fruit (avoid those sprayed in sulphur dioxide, however) instead of cakes and biscuits. They will provide you with more nutrients and long-lasting energy, and will keep your blood sugar level stable.
- You eat butter rather than margarine or spread. Butter is full of vitamin D, whereas margarine often contains hydrogenated fats. And butter tastes better!
- You eat rye or wholegrain bread (complex carbohydrate).
- You drink organic milk, which is richer in omega-3 fatty acids than normal milk .
- You drink herbal teas rather than coffee or tea.

questionnaire: **healthy eating**

By the end of this step you will have a good idea as to whether or not your diet is having a **positive or negative** effect on your fertility as well as your general health. Answer these questions then re-read the parts of the step that **relate to the areas** where you feel your diet needs some reconsideration and could **benefit from change**

 1 Do you eat less than five portions of fruit or vegetables per day?
yes ☐ **no** ☐
You need the essential nutrients that these provide in order to nourish your body.

2 Do you often skip breakfast?
yes ☐ **no** ☐
This is the most important meal of the day, especially for women, as skipping breakfast will imbalance your blood sugar level and your hormones (see page 102).

3 Do you ever skip lunch or dinner?
yes ☐ **no** ☐
Skipping a meal will trick your body into thinking it is being starved, and it will tend to stockpile glucose and lay it down as fat. Your blood sugar level will also drop and this could affect your hormonal balance.

4 Do you regularly crave sugary foods?
yes ☐ **no** ☐
Your blood sugar levels need rebalancing. See pages 102–103 to make sure you know how to do this.

5 Do you drink more than two cups of coffee (or 4–5 cups of tea) a day?
yes ☐ **no** ☐
Caffeine has a diuretic effect on the body, and robs it of essential fluids (see page 108).

 6 Do you usually eat white bread?
yes ☐ **no** ☐
White bread, along with other forms of refined carbohydrates, is not very nourishing. You will get more energy and fewer sugar cravings if you reduce or cut these out of your diet, and consume instead complex carbs such as brown bread and brown rice (see page 102).

7 Do you often add salt to food once it has been cooked?
yes ☐ **no** ☐
Salt is bad for blood pressure and it is important to cut down on intake. Read page 107 for ways in which to do this.

8 Do you eat processed convenience foods or takeaways more than once a week?
yes ☐ **no** ☐
Ideally, you should cut these out of your diet altogether, but if you do consume them, limit them as much as possible. They are invariably high in salt, fats, and/or additives.

 9 Do you suffer from poor digestion and/or constipation?
yes ☐ **no** ☐
Your body could be having trouble absorbing all the nutrients you are eating (see pages 110–111).

10 Do you usually have dinner less than 2 hours before going to bed?

yes ☐   no ☐

This affects digestion. Try to eat earlier and more lightly so that digestion improves.

11 Do you always finish what is on your plate, even if you are no longer hungry?

yes ☐   no ☐

You are more likely to gain excess weight and may find you suffer from bloating, flatulence, and/or heartburn. Stop when your body tells you you have had enough to eat and you will feel better and in control.

12 Do you regularly snack on sugary or salty/fatty foods?

yes ☐   no ☐

Try to find alternative, healthier snacks to avoid putting on weight and unbalancing your blood sugar levels.

13 Do you drink less than 1 litre (2.2 pints) of water a day, excluding teas and coffees?

yes ☐   no ☐

Dehydration can cause blood sugar imbalance and a feeling of tiredness, which can make you overeat to compensate for the lack of energy.

14 Do you binge eat?

yes ☐   no ☐

This will cause your hormones and blood sugar levels to yo-yo and could impact on your chances of getting pregnant. See pages 111–112 for ways to avoid this.

15 Are you constantly dieting?

yes ☐   no ☐

Again, this will affect the balance of your hormones and could affect your fertility. Aim for a healthy, sensible, and realistic diet. Re-read this step so that you can try to follow the advice more closely.

your**score**

0–3 No one is an angel when it comes to food, but you don't seem to be far from being one. This is one area of your life where you are already doing the best you can to boost your fertility.

4–7 You are eating reasonably well, on the whole. You should nonetheless assess your "yes" answers to see where you can improve your dietary habits, just to make sure that they are not affecting your chances of conceiving.

8–11 You probably struggle to eat healthily. This could in part be due to lifestyle factors, such as working long hours, which are also affecting your diet. Re-read Steps 5 and 6 to see how you can improve both. Make changes over a period of time and you will see a steady improvement.

12–15 You don't need me to tell you that you eat unhealthily! You may be deficient in several essential nutrients and have regular problems with blood sugar levels. Your hormonal balance is probably also affected. Fortunately, diet is one of the easiest factors in fertility to improve, so start to find ways of changing your eating habits. Your health will doubtless quickly reap the benefit, as could your chances of conception.

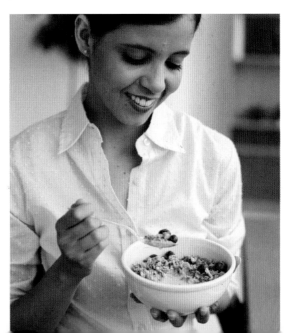

Our **emotional** and **physical** selves are intrinsically linked: making time for yourself to **relax** and **unwind** can **boost fertility**

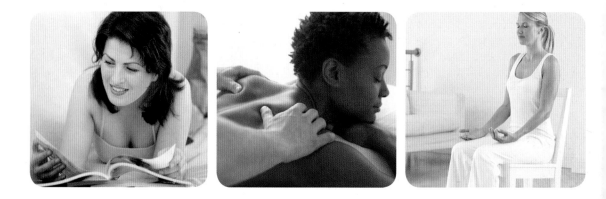

step**seven**
the mind–body link

Your questions answered on:

step seven: the mind–body link

The **role the mind plays** in fertility and conception is still not clearly understood, but there does appear to be a link. What **type of personality** you are, your **ability to cope with stress**, your **past experiences**: these are just some of the many psychological factors that influence the way your body functions

Q What is the mind–body link?

For me, the mind–body link is not just about the influence that emotions have on our physical processes. It is also about being able to listen to ourselves, about being fully in tune with our bodies, and using that awareness to influence how we live and how we feel. It means being in control of our physical and mental state so that we can manage our lives on a day-to-day basis as well as possible.

Stress is something that exists in all our lives. It has always been present and human beings are designed to be able to deal with it, thanks to their nervous system and the fight–flight system of response (see pages 82–83). Problems arise when the stress response fails and symptoms of stress begin to manifest themselves. It is therefore how you deal with stress and other negative emotions that matters, not whether stress is or isn't present in your life. And I firmly believe that you can choose to handle stress, through relaxation, through your lifestyle (including exercise and diet), and through building up your reserves. These three elements are key to getting the balance back in your life and to feeling good. By achieving both physical and emotional well-being, I truly believe you can improve your fertility.

When you are trying for a baby, it is vital to find ways to relax when faced with stress and to get the blood flowing to the organs where it is needed, such as the ovaries, the other reproductive organs, and the brain. You may need to learn relaxation techniques, including breathing and meditation (see pages 122–123). You may also need to slow down and to rest more. The result will be a slower heart rate, better blood flow, a feeling of being more relaxed and in control, and a more positive mood.

Q Can your personality type affect your fertility?

There are many different personality types and, of course, most people are a combination of more than one. For example, you can be an optimist, a pessimist, a perfectionist, a fatalist, or a mixture of all of these, depending on the day or on the circumstances. Most of us have a predominant emotion and this is fine if yours is generally positive but more problematic if you are predominantly angry, worried, fearful, or weighed down by grief. It is important to work out if your dominant emotion is blocking your ability to get things done in life, including getting pregnant.

If you constantly think negatively, for example, you may become afraid of everything. Molehills quickly become insurmountable mountains; life becomes very complicated and stressful and, before long, everything becomes difficult. You need to work this through, using the advice in this step to help you, because this could be affecting your ability to relax and, ultimately, even your fertility. I believe that emotions are inextricably linked to how our bodies function, and for that reason, it is important to try to understand and deal with the many different facets of your personality and how you handle your emotions.

Zita's **tip**

Practise looking at life **from a positive perspective** to improve your overall sense of well-being.

Q Can emotions block fertility?

I believe that negative emotions such as fear, anxiety, and grief can all impact on the chances of conception. Emotions such as these cause raised levels of stress hormones (see pages 82–84), which can interfere with the immune system, hormonal balance, and, as a result, fertility. Western medicine, which is largely evidence-based and relies on scientifically approved studies, has not yet fully understood the complex interplay between stress, emotions, and fertility, although it is starting to recognize that there seems to be a link. Yet Chinese medicine (see pages 133–134) has long recognized the relationship between the mental and the physical: the belief being that the meridian system that runs through the body is affected by different emotions such as the ones above, and these can cause blockages within the system that lead to physical problems.

Q Which emotions are likely to have a detrimental effect?

When I ask the women I treat how they feel emotionally, the most common responses are that they feel worried or afraid, frustrated, angry, jealous, sad, or depressed. While it is not (yet) possible to prove that these emotions can block conception, it does appear that there is sometimes a link, based on my experience of the couples I see. This connection may be due to the physical effects of stress (such as a disrupted hormonal balance).

Fear and worry are common. Sometimes the woman is afraid of getting pregnant (she may not be psychologically ready), but more often she is worried that it may never happen. These emotions can lead to her developing symptoms of depression and stress and to having a negative view of everything connected with pregnancy. She can become low on every level and lacking in energy.

Anger, frustration, and jealousy can manifest themselves verbally or physically. In the latter case, the woman

shortens her breath and breathes more shallowly. Her heart rate goes up and production of stress hormones increases. If she bottles up those feelings, she can start to get tension in her back, neck, and shoulders, and/or to suffer from headaches.

Sadness and grief are also very common. Sadness can be caused by the inability to get pregnant, and this can lead to depression, or it can be caused by grief for a previous loss: either a miscarriage or a termination. Also the loss of a parent is often a source of much conscious or unconscious grief.

Q I'm not coping with my feelings. How can I get help with my negative emotions?

If you are currently experiencing one or several negative emotions such as the ones described above, you need to work on ways to change your thoughts so that they play a less dominant role in your emotions. I realize this is not easy and cannot happen overnight, but you need to find the source of the emotions and the best way for you to manage it. This might involve a combination of relaxation techniques (see page 122), talking to someone close to you (not necessarily your partner), making certain lifestyle changes, including doing regular exercise and getting plenty of sleep, and counselling or perhaps psychotherapy.

By adopting one or several of the above methods, you will feel you are taking control of these negative emotions and this will enable you to feel less dominated by them, thereby reducing their impact on your well-being.

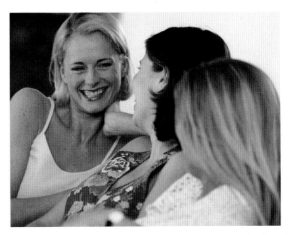

It helps to be optimistic and outgoing because your predominant state of mind has underlying effects on your health and well-being.

Q Is past emotional or physical trauma a factor in a person's fertility?

Clients I see who have had major childhood traumas can have psychological difficulty with the idea of getting pregnant, however much they want to conceive. It is not uncommon, for example, for men or women who suffered from a serious illness in childhood to expect to have trouble conceiving, even though their past illness has nothing to do with their fertility.

Similarly, women I see who have lost one or both parents in their childhood (especially their mother) and who have been deeply marked by their loss are sometimes stuck in their grief. They may have a subconscious fear of getting pregnant and of subsequently dying, or they may be frightened at the thought of parenting, having prematurely lost their own parenting role model. Whatever the reason, they may not be consciously aware that they have not grieved properly for their parent, and may need counselling or therapy to "free" themselves and allow their lives to move on.

It goes without saying that anyone who has suffered sexual, physical, or emotional abuse as a child may have been profoundly affected by this and may find this impacts on their fertility unless they seek appropriate professional help. Similarly, a previous abusive relationship in adulthood can cause lasting damage to a person's emotional stability and affect their future relationships. It is important to try to deal with these situations if you think they could be affecting your psychological and physical well-being, as they could end up impacting on your ability to conceive.

Q Can the way a person was parented affect their fertility?

The majority of people were parented in a way that would not affect their own chances of becoming parents. However, it can happen that some people have or had difficult relationships with one or both parents and this could subconsciously be affecting their chances of getting pregnant. For example, I have seen clients who are no longer on speaking terms with their parents, or who feel constantly undermined by one or both of them; if their parents divorced this can also lead to a psychological blockage at the idea of becoming a parent. On a similarly anecdotal level, but one which I feel is also significant, a lot of the women I see who were adopted seem to think

that they will be unable to have their own child and will end up adopting. If there is no medical foundation for their belief, these women need to consult a professional who can help them to see beyond their anxieties before they start to dominate their emotions and hinder their chances of conceiving.

It may be that your situation is not dissimilar to one of those described above, in which case it is worth considering whether this could be affecting you in ways that you had not previously understood. If this is the case, you need to seek professional help with a suitably trained counsellor or psychotherapist to help clarify some of the issues you might have surrounding parenting. But I always tell clients that they shouldn't have to dig too deep to find the reasons.

Q Can relationship worries have an effect?

Although problems linked to your past can, in my view, impact on fertility, those linked to your current relationship can also have a similar effect. You may be very aware of the problems but have such a strong desire for a baby that you are pushing aside difficult issues surrounding your relationship. However, this in itself could be causing an unnecessary amount of stress in your system and a psychological blockage concerning conception.

Similarly, some women have doubts – which may be conscious or not – about their partner's ability to be a good father to their child. This could be because of the way he himself was parented, or because of his personality, or even his job (for example, if he works unsocial hours, is away for long periods of time, or is not financially secure). Alternatively, a couple might not share the same views about how to raise a child. Either way, the woman might have some concerns about her choice of partner, but is willing to set these aside while she tries to get pregnant.

It is also quite common for one partner to be keener than the other to start a family, and this too can lead to pressure and tension in a relationship. It may be, for example, that the male partner does not feel ready to start a family, perhaps because he considers himself to be too young, or because he already has children from a previous relationship, but as a result, the woman starts to be affected psychologically by her partner's reluctance.

There are no quick fixes to problems such as these but bringing them out in the open so they can be discussed and resolved will help to minimize any damage to your relationship and to your plans to have a baby together.

find out more: **are we ready for a baby?**

You will most certainly answer a resounding "yes" to this question because, after all, you have bought this book and are actively seeking ways to improve your chances of conceiving a baby. But at this point I would like you to reflect on why you are trying to have a baby.

It's quite common for couples to try to conceive because the time is right in their careers (or simply because they don't have much time left, if the woman is over 35), or because "all their friends" are having babies and they don't want to feel left out. They may feel overly frustrated if a baby doesn't happen straight away because they are used to controlling all other aspects of their lives; or may be trying to time conception to fit in with a moment when the house is purchased and decorated and everything is in its place. There is nothing inherently wrong with any of these reasons, except for the fact that the reality of what a baby will mean is often strangely absent. Conception is not an end but a beginning and I urge couples to look beyond it and consider how they will make space in their lives when a child becomes a reality.

why do you **want a child**?

- Are all your friends having babies?
- Are you under pressure from a partner or family?
- Do you want a way out of your job?
- Is now the right time in your career?
- Are you in a good relationship, and feel you will make great parents?

imagine what life will be like…

I find that many of the couples I see – and women in particular – like the romantic image of motherhood but tend to blank out the 24-hour care of a helpless newborn and the inevitable complications that children bring to life, even though the rewards are many. Paradoxically, there are as many people who are completely unable to see the positives. Having a baby seems to be the right thing to do but all they see is the negative side: restricted finances and independence, a curtailed social and sex life, and sleep deprivation for years to come. They may be secretly afraid of what pregnancy and, more importantly, parenthood will bring. If this is how you feel, you need to discuss your misgivings openly and honestly with your partner and make a conscious decision to find out more about how rewarding parenthood can be, whatever the difficulties and sacrifices involved. Hopefully, you will then feel you have made the right decision to try to get pregnant and be calmer and more prepared for what awaits you. I believe that being in the right frame of mind for parenthood will help you conceive.

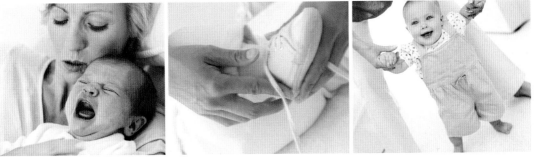

There are times when every parent struggles and feels unable to cope.

Looking after a baby means taking care of his or her every need.

But the rewards are invariably rich as you watch your baby grow and develop.

find out more: **learning to relax**

I am convinced that **finding an inner tranquillity** and **relaxation**, and being able to do so on a daily basis, is essential for **maintaining health and well-being**.

Some of the main self-help relaxation techniques are included here – you will soon discover which one works best for you. However, whichever you choose, you will find your way of breathing is key to its success. Many people breathe shallowly, using their chest rather than their diaphragm (the dome-shaped muscle at the base of the lungs), with the result that the lungs are not fully utilized and the body does not receive as much oxygen as it should. In times of tension or stress you may breathe so quickly and shallowly that you become short of breath and light-headed.

Boost **oxygen intake** by as much as

30%

by maintaining good posture. This opens up your chest cavity making more energy available for your mind and muscles.

learning to breathe

Although it seems absurd to have to practise something you do automatically, learning to breathe more slowly and deeply will reduce muscle tension in your neck and chest, decrease the energy required to breathe, and improve your circulation and overall physical health.

Deep breathing exercise

▢ Lie on your back with your knees bent. (If this feels uncomfortable place a pillow under your knees.) Place one hand on your upper chest and the other just below your rib cage. This helps you to monitor your chest and to feel your diaphragm move as you breathe.

▢ Close your eyes and breathe in slowly through your nose so that your stomach moves out against your lower hand. The upper hand should remain as still as possible.
▢ Tighten your stomach muscles, letting them fall inwards as you exhale through pursed lips. Your upper hand should continue to remain as still as possible.

Practise this exercise for 5 to 10 minutes, twice a day. You may find it is rather tiring at first, but it will become easier and will eventually become automatic. Once you are used to breathing like this, practise while sitting in a chair, with your head and neck relaxed and supported, and your legs bent and in front of you.

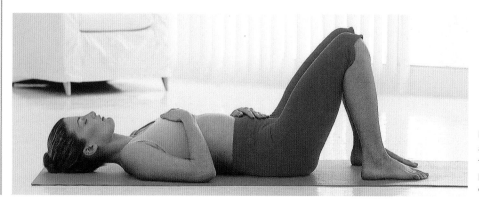

Practise breathing in a mindful and focused way to promote feelings of well-being.

visualization

Once you have learnt to breathe deeply, you can try visualization as a relaxation method. This involves closing your eyes and focusing your mind on whatever setting you find most relaxing: for example, this might be an idyllic beach with water lapping at your feet and the sun warming your skin. Whatever you choose, picture the scene, imagine the sounds, the sensations on your skin, even the smells that you might expect. After a while, you will find that you have cleared your mind of all but the most pleasurable sensations, and that your body has reached a level of deep relaxation and of slow, regular breathing. Some people find that a CD or tape helps them to do this.

Whatever you choose to visualize, make sure you repeat the technique on a daily basis for 20 minutes. Allow only positive thoughts into your head. Hypnotherapy is another route to this type of relaxation (see page 133).

Some people believe that our bodies are very receptive to positive thoughts and that this can benefit our health. By imagining a positive outcome to a particular situation, they believe it is possible to reduce stress, improve overall well-being, and therefore to boost fertility. Once you have reached a relaxed physical state, you can start to send positive thoughts to every part of your body, focusing on your reproductive organs and their fertility, and visualizing exactly what you want your body to achieve, such as your ovaries releasing a ripe and healthy egg. I use this technique when helping couples to visualize an embryo implanting in the womb following IVF treatment.

progressive **muscle relaxation**

This technique teaches you to recognize the tension or stress in your body by purposefully creating and releasing tension, starting at one end of your body and finishing at the other. By noticing tension in different parts of the body, we gain awareness of when we feel tense or relaxed.

meditation

There are many different forms of meditation, which in essence is a way of achieving a deep state of relaxation through breathing. There is much scientific evidence for the physical and psychological benefits of this relaxation technique, which include a drop in heart rate and in the production of stress hormones. It works at a deep level on the parasympathetic and sympathetic nervous systems (see page 82), helping to rebalance them so that the parasympathetic is able to function more effectively.

Transcendental meditation (TM) and Acem meditation are two of the more popular forms. The TM technique is practiced for 20 minutes twice a day while sitting with your eyes closed, enabling your mind to "transcend" to a quieter state. Acem meditation allows you to have thoughts coming into your head, to accept them, then to let them float off while you repeat a sound that you are given. After meditation, your body and brain feel energized once more.

Meditation needs to be learned, but this does not take long. Afterwards, it is easy to practise it at home. You simply need to find somewhere warm, quiet, and comfortable to lie or sit, and to set aside time each day to practise.

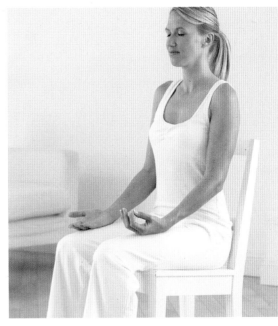

Daily meditation involves a simple technique that allows the mind and body to rest and releases mental and physical stress.

Q Can fears about pregnancy and childbirth have a negative effect?

Some women have a genuine fear of pregnancy and childbirth. I often see women who have had one child and experienced a bad labour and birth and this has an impact on their trying for a second child. Alternatively, for women who are used to controlling how they look through diet and exercise, the thought of this loss of control over their body can be genuinely terrifying, with ongoing effects on their chances of conceiving.

A fear of childbirth is also a factor in some women's psychological well-being and it can influence their ability to get pregnant. They might dread the loss of control over their body during labour or worry that they might not be able to manage the pain; they might also be very frightened of the (perceived) risks involved in giving birth. Perhaps they know someone who had a terrible experience of childbirth – indeed, it is sometimes hard for women to avoid hearing horror stories of childbirth from friends, family, and colleagues – and this may have coloured their judgement of how much they want to put themselves through the experience.

The same can happen to men: they can be made to panic at the thought of seeing their partner in severe pain, and their baby "in danger" during the birth. Secretly, many men do not relish the thought of being present during their partner's labour and the thought of having to go through this rite of passage could affect their desire for parenthood.

If you feel you are developing a fear of pregnancy or childbirth, you should attempt to inform yourself as much as possible through books and properly researched statistics on the internet, rather than speaking to doom-monger friends. You can then understand the relative and very small risks of things going wrong.

As for dreading the loss of your pre-pregnancy body, by eating sensibly (rather than "for two", which is unnecessary) and exercising regularly during pregnancy, most women find that they lose all their pregnancy weight within a short time of giving birth and that the changes to their bodies are imperceptible to anyone other than themselves. Even their partners do not necessarily notice. And in my experience, once women find themselves with a wonderful new baby, this more than compensates for any minor physical changes.

Q What other issues can influence the mind–body link?

Some women – and men too – can put additional pressures on themselves and these could be influencing their ability to get pregnant. For example, they may be desperate to get pregnant within a specific time-frame, or to have a boy rather than a girl (or vice versa); or they may have to cope with family and friends making unhelpful comments along the lines of "When are you going to have a baby?" and "When am I going to be a grandmother?" Anything that puts extra pressure on someone to conceive can be detrimental to their mental and physical well-being, unless that person knows how to manage the comments and the expectations.

If you think you are suffering from self-imposed or external pressures of the sort described above, it is vital that you find ways of coping with them. Humour or firmness (or both) may be necessary to deflect other people's comments, which are usually made unthinkingly but without malice. You may prefer to explain the situation to them, or you may, on the contrary, prefer to stay vague about your plans, while making it clear that you don't appreciate such prying into your life. Only you will know how you wish to handle this sensitive area and the way in which you do it will vary depending on who you are, and who you are dealing with. But it is important that you decide on a strategy, as this will help you to handle these external pressures. One thing I would add, however, is that it is better to deal with the situation than to cut friends and family out of your social life because this will restrict you on every level.

When it comes to self-imposed pressures, you need to analyse and understand why that particular issue is so important to you, and then to imagine what would happen if – worst case scenario – you did not get your wish. If necessary, seek help from a counsellor, and consider the benefits of relaxation exercises (see pages 122–123) in order to reduce tension and stress.

> ## Zita's **tip**
> Feeling **in control of your life** and thoughts means working out what you **need to change**.

Q I'm finding it hard to cope with other people's pregnancies. Is this normal?

When you have been trying to get pregnant for a while, one of the hardest situations to have to cope with, and one which causes a lot of external stress, is finding out that a close friend or relative is expecting a baby. Hearing that this person has achieved what you most want at the moment – a pregnancy – can bring to the surface many negative emotions, such as sadness, envy, and anger, and these can be very difficult to control. If this is the case, try to remind yourself that the fact that this person is having a baby does not reduce the chances of you getting pregnant. There is not a finite amount of babies "to be had", so someone else's pregnancy has no impact on your fertility. It may help to be honest with that person and explain to them why you are currently finding it difficult to rejoice at their news.

Q Is it OK to talk to someone other than my partner about how I am feeling?

Many women (and men) find it helpful if they can off-load their anxieties and stress onto one or two trusted people who aren't their partner. That person could be a close friend or a family member, or a professional counsellor who is neutral and has no emotional link. The important thing is that this person can act as a release valve for you, because however good your relationship with your partner might be, it is not always helpful to either of you if you confide solely in each other. Indeed, if your partner is your only outlet for your concerns, you may be placing an emotional burden that is too heavy for him or her to carry alone. You therefore might benefit from talking to someone else, in confidence and on a regular basis.

find out more: **the simple things**

It seems obvious, but all too often people do not even find time for the most basic form of relaxation: doing nothing. There seems to be a perception nowadays that we always have to be buzzing around "doing something". Our lives and work mean that we are often very busy, but I feel that many of us end up running almost "on empty". We have very few reserves in the tank, and when you are trying for a baby, particularly if you have been trying for a little while, it is vital that you build up those reserves. That means getting a balance in your life between your daily, frenetic lifestyle and having time out when you truly relax.

simple ways **to relax**

- Listening to music that makes you feel calm.
- Sitting in a park or garden listening to bird song.
- Getting your partner to massage you with aromatherapy oils that are good for relaxation, such as lavender, orange, and camomile.
- Lighting candles with delicious scents such as rose, orange sandalwood, or ylang ylang, to help create a wonderfully relaxing atmosphere in a room.

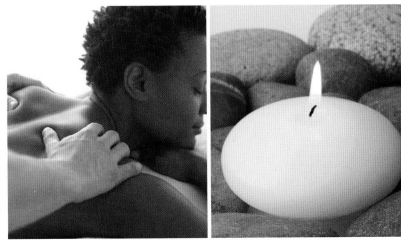

Massaging your partner with aromatic oils is both relaxing and highly sensual.

Lighting scented candles in a dimly lit room creates a relaxing and soothing atmosphere.

questionnaire: **emotional health**

Having read this step you will have a clearer idea as to whether or not **psychological and emotional factors** in your life are having an effect on **your general health** and therefore your **chances of conceiving**. Answer these questions, scoring 1 for every "yes", then check my summary of how your emotional balance is faring

1 Do you like to control your life rather than leave things to chance?
yes ☐ **no** ☐
Not managing to conceive as planned could be causing you unwanted stress. Read pages 122–123 to learn more about relaxation techniques.

2 Do you find it hard to do nothing?
yes ☐ **no** ☐
It is important to have a balance in your life and to build up your reserves. Read page 125 to learn more about simple ways to relax.

3 Is your glass usually half empty?
yes ☐ **no** ☐
Pessimism can lead to negativity. Consider finding ways (including relaxation techniques and therapy) that could help you to see things more positively, as this is important when trying to get pregnant.

4 Do you have any concerns about your partner's ability to be a good parent?
yes ☐ **no** ☐
Different views about how to raise a child can put a strain on a relationship. If this is the case for you, you should openly discuss the issues with your partner sooner rather than later.

5 Do you currently have a difficult relationship with either, or both, of your parents?
yes ☐ **no** ☐
Outstanding issues within your family could be affecting your desire to become a parent. Read page 120 to find out ways to address your feelings and work things through.

6 Did you suffer the loss of a parent as a child?
yes ☐ **no** ☐
Unresolved grief could be affecting you. You may have a subconscious or conscious fear of parenting because your own family life is associated with loss and sadness. Ask yourself whether you need to seek professional help in order to deal with your situation (see page 119).

7 Have you suffered any other significant losses in your family, or feel you are still being affected by a past pregnancy loss such as a miscarriage or a termination?
yes ☐ **no** ☐
Grieving can be a lengthy process and you may not have given yourself time to mourn sufficiently and move on from your loss. This may be having an impact on your ability to let go. A period of counselling may help.

8 Are you worried that you may not be able to conceive within a particular time-frame that feels important to you?

yes ☐ **no** ☐

Self-imposed pressures of this sort can raise stress levels and this could impact on your chances of conceiving. See page 124 to find ways of learning to cope with and manage your expectations.

9 Are you being asked regularly when you are going to get pregnant or feel under pressure to produce a first grandchild?

yes ☐ **no** ☐

External pressures are never helpful, however well-meant. See page 124 for advice on how to cope and how to stay relaxed.

10 Were you adopted as a child?

yes ☐ **no** ☐

Women who were adopted sometimes have a deep-rooted feeling that they are more likely to fail to conceive and will end up adopting too (see page 120).

11 Are you frightened about the prospect of going through a pregnancy and/or labour?

yes ☐ **no** ☐

Excessive anxiety about the physical aspect of giving birth could be impacting on your chances of conceiving. Read about safe, normal deliveries and don't listen to scare stories.

12 Do you wonder how you will make room in your life for a baby?

yes ☐ **no** ☐

Some couples who are tryng to get pregnant are privately worried about loss of freedom and other negative aspects of having a child. Read page 121 for advice on how to reassure yourselves.

your**score**

0–2 You probably have a reasonably healthy emotional balance when it comes to the idea of getting pregnant. However, you should not ignore any of your "yes" answers, and make sure that they do not impact in any way on the mind–body element in pregnancy.

3–5 Analyse your "yes" answers and work on improving those areas that could be affecting you psychologically and therefore physically. Find ways of relaxing on a regular basis.

6–8 You should consider seeking professional help to work on the various areas that could be affecting your ability to conceive. Re-read this step, learn a good relaxation technique, and read Step 8 on complementary therapies as well.

9–12 Now you have read this step you have probably realized that your state of mind could be affecting your fertility. Seek professional help now – it could take a few months for any benefit to be felt – to ensure that your health is not compromised by any psychological and relationship issues. Find ways to help yourself in this step and in Step 8.

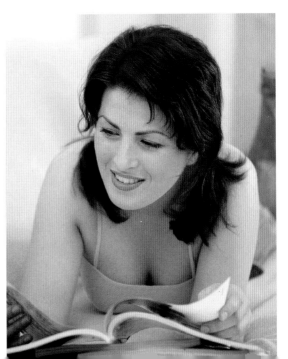

The **key to success** with any complementary therapy is finding a **practitioner** with whom you feel **comfortable**

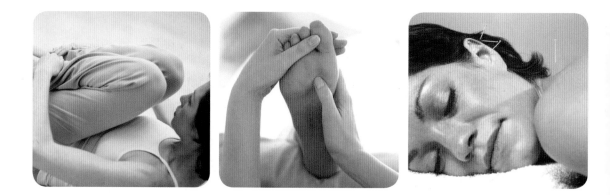

step**eight**
complementary therapies

Your questions answered on:

step eight: **complementary therapies**

I believe in an **integrated approach** to health, and therefore to getting pregnant. This means making the most of both **complementary** and **mainstream medicine**. Women who are trying to get pregnant can get a great deal out of complementary therapies, and this step offers advice on **which can be of help**

Q What is the difference between complementary and alternative medicine?

The couples I see are often not sure how to refer to non-conventional forms of medicine or treatment. In essence, complementary medicine covers those therapies which, as their name suggests, complement a diagnosis or treatment from conventional medicine. They do not themselves cover diagnosis, and they simply complement mainstream medical practice. Alternative medicine refers to those therapies that offer an alternative system of diagnosis and treatment to conventional medicine.

Q What are the benefits of an integrated approach to medicine?

An integrated approach to medicine involves working with both Western medicine and with complementary therapies, and combining them so that they suit your needs. One of the advantages of complementary therapies is that they enable the patient to be listened to properly. People can spend uninterrupted time talking to the practitioner without feeling that they

Zita's **tip**

> Combine **mainstream medicine** with **complementary therapies** to get the best of both worlds.

are part of a fast-moving conveyor belt. Sadly, nowadays, GPs are so overworked that the average consultation lasts only around seven minutes, and this is not conducive to establishing a good patient–carer relationship, nor to getting to the bottom of any health situation that is at all complex. Very often, when you are planning to have a baby, you are a bit anxious, especially if you have been trying for a while, and it is dispiriting to feel you have to get your point across in a matter of minutes. It can cause emotions to be bottled up and problems to be stored away for far too long. Making use of complementary or alternative medicine (CAM) can be a good way of managing anxiety and stress and of enabling you to feel you are actively contributing to your well-being. It allows you to feel in control of the situation.

Q What shall I do if my GP is not keen on complementary therapies?

I feel GPs need to be more open to the evidence available. I still come across many GPs and hospital consultants who are very sceptical of the benefits of complementary and alternative therapies, in any shape or form. As far as they are concerned, Western medicine offers the only answers to health problems. It is therefore hard when a woman believes in and wants to try a particular treatment and goes to see her doctor, to be met only by negativity, simply because there is no significant trial-based scientific evidence to support the alleged benefits of the treatment. The woman, who wants to be proactive in her attempt to improve her chances of conception, leaves demoralized because she does not have the support of her GP or specialist.

If this happens to you, my advice is to inform yourself as much as possible about the therapy you are proposing to begin, so that you find out if there is evidence of its benefits. There is increasing evidence to show that some – but not all – complementary and alternative medicines can help with fertility and other areas of health, and this is crucial when you are trying to decide which therapy to try. You might even find that, as a result of your research, your doctor becomes more supportive of your combined approach to your healthcare. Remember, I see things from both sides and very often GPs do come across therapists who talk a great deal of psychobabble with little demonstrable effect.

Q How can I find the right therapy?

Finding your way through the jungle of therapies and therapists can be a daunting, confusing, and time-consuming task. Most importantly, I would advise you to do your research. Find out which therapies suit you best in terms of what they offer, how convenient they are for your lifestyle and where you live/work, which ones are good for the specific issue(s) you want to deal with, and which ones you can afford. Ask around, speak to friends and colleagues. Personal recommendation is always valuable, as are recommendations to avoid a particular therapy or practitioner! Use the internet to research the facts and figures and speak to the regulatory bodies of any therapies that interest you.

It is important not to use the scatter-gun approach. Avoid signing up to too many therapies. Once you think you have narrowed down the options, you need to find a practitioner, if you have not already been recommended one. It is important to establish that he or she is contracted to a regulatory body or authority (see page 132).

Q Are all complementary therapies beneficial for fertility?

I believe that some therapies can be beneficial to people who are trying to conceive, even though there may not be much, or any, scientific evidence to prove this. The therapies I offer in my clinic include:
- hypnotherapy (see page 133)
- Pilates

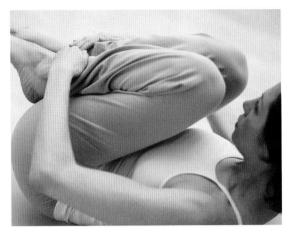

Pilates exercises improve fertility as they help reduce stress and therefore restore the hormonal balance of the body.

- Traditional Chinese Medicine (TCM) (see page 133) and acupuncture (see pages 134–135)
- manual lymphatic drainage (see page 137)
- reflexology (see page 137)
- visualization (see page 123)
- nutritional therapy (using food and supplements to encourage the body's natural healing)
- massage.

Most importantly, at my clinic we offer a plan of action based on a questionnaire that pinpoints what you need to do to help you to get pregnant.

The fact that I offer only the therapies above does not mean that I believe others are of no help for fertility. However, I think you should be careful if using Chinese or any other type of herbal medicine, unless you are working with a registered practitioner, because of the risk of harmful interaction between the treatment and either your diet, any prescription medicines you might be taking, or even just your body's natural processes. Many herbs have interactions with medications and can disrupt your hormones, so just because something is herbal and therefore "natural" it doesn't necessarily mean it is safe.

Q What should I do first?

Once you have researched what the benefits are of a particular therapy and found a potential practitioner, go and talk to him or her before you sign up to any course of treatment. My golden rule is that you should feel comfortable with that person. The patient–practitioner relationship is, I believe, key to the success of a complementary therapy. If you feel that the therapist talks more about himself or herself than about you or is putting pressure on you to commit to treatment, or if you simply don't "click" with that person, then treatment may not be as effective for you. I am a firm believer in gut feeling; it is easy to want to believe everything you are told, but give yourself a little time to reflect before making a final choice

of therapy and practitioner. Keep in mind that even though one treatment works for one individual, it may not work for another.

Don't sign up for a long course of treatments and don't flit from one treatment to another, trying one then moving on before you have had a chance to see if it works. That said, it is also important that you set yourself a time-frame for treatment: you should not be going week after

Q Are **complementary therapies** regulated?

Complementary and alternative medicine (CAM) as a whole is moving towards organizing itself into clear professional regulated bodies, so that people know what they are getting when they seek out a particular practitioner. There are two categories of regulation:

Statutory regulation is recommended for therapies where there is perceived to be a significant risk to the public from poor practice. Currently, both osteopathy and chiropractic techniques have statutory regulation, which means that by law practitioners have to join the register of their regulatory bodies (see Resources, page 183), otherwise it is illegal for them to practise. Acupuncture (through the British Acupuncture Council) and herbal medicine are also likely to have statutory regulation in the near future.

Voluntary self-regulation is chosen by most complementary therapists. This means that they belong to a single, professional body that registers its practitioners. But such bodies cannot force practitioners to register, and the standards required by them can vary, as can the standards of such individual practitioners. A practitioner registered with one of these bodies is not guaranteed to have a high level of knowledge or skill, but any practitioner who is not even registered with the relevant professional body should be avoided. Most complementary therapy bodies have worked closely with the Foundation for Integrated Health (see Resources, page 183) in recent years to raise standards.

A House of Lords Select Committee report divided CAM into three groups (see table below).

complementary and alternative medicine groups	
Group	**CAMs covered**
Professionally organized alternative therapies	Chiropractic techniques, osteopathy (both of these have statutory regulation), herbal medicine, homeopathy, acupuncture.
Complementary therapies	Alexander technique, aromatherapy, Bach and other flower remedies, body work therapies (including massage), counselling, stress therapy, hypnotherapy, meditation, reflexology, shiatsu, healing (including Reiki), Maharishi Ayurvedic medicine, nutritional medicine, yoga.
Alternative disciplines	*Long-established and traditional systems of healthcare:* anthroposophical medicine, Ayurvedic medicine, Chinese herbal medicine, Eastern medicine, naturopathy, Traditional Chinese Medicine (TCM) *Other alternative disciplines:* crystal therapy, dowsing, iridology, kinesiology, radionics.

week, year after year, without any visible signs of success. If you are trying for a baby, give yourself four to six months, then review the situation to see whether any improvements have been made.

The reason that complementary therapies are sometimes successful is that they look at the whole person (or couple) on every level: emotionally, physically, and at what else is happening in their lives – their relationship, finances, and stresses – no matter how trivial. It is important to be able to make changes outside the treatment to bring the relevant areas of your life back into balance.

Q Is hypnotherapy useful for fertility?

Hypnotherapy is a deep form of relaxation that can benefit your psychological and physical health. Contrary to many people's assumptions, it can only work with the patient's consent, and at no time does he or she lose control. During hypnotherapy, the conscious part of your brain is temporarily switched off and the subconscious part comes to the surface. In this state, you are receptive to suggestion and can be desensitized for negative thoughts, deep-rooted fears, and phobias.

Hypnotherapy also reduces the impact of stress, so it can be particularly beneficial if you are still suffering as a result of a past event, such as a miscarriage or termination of pregnancy. It can also be helpful if you are suffering from unexplained infertility or performance anxiety (in men) as it can remove subconscious mental blocks that could be getting in the way of you conceiving. Even if you do not manage to relax enough to enter a meditative state (although most people can), a hypnotherapist will teach you to relax sufficiently so that positive images and thoughts can come to the forefront of your mind. As a result, negative thoughts and emotions can be pushed aside, which improves self-confidence and self-esteem.

Once you have been taught how to reach this relaxed state by a therapist, you will be able to do this at home, so it need not be an expensive form of therapy. It can also be combined with visualization and affirmation techniques, to give you a more positive outlook on your life in general and on your fertility in particular, and this could be just what you need to boost your chances of conceiving.

Q What is Traditional Chinese Medicine (TCM)?

In Chinese medicine, there are certain rules for living life within natural laws. The belief is that our health is governed by a vital life force, known as *qi* (pronounced "chee"), which flows through certain invisible pathways called meridians. Most of the principal meridians are named after the major internal organs through which they pass. TCM takes a holistic view of disease, treating the body as a whole. When the *qi* becomes unbalanced, illness develops. Symptoms indicate an imbalance in the meridian of one or more organs. Each organ displays a specific pattern of disharmony that the practitioner diagnoses through observation and analysis of symptoms.

Treatment is provided to restore the flow of *qi* and thereby restore the body's balance. TCM uses different forms of treatment including herbal medicine, massage, and acupuncture. I do not use or advise patients to use herbal medicine, because of a possible adverse drug–nutrient interaction. I do, however, use acupuncture and massage, both of which I believe can help a woman who is trying to conceive.

before you start

When thinking about using a particular form of complementary therapy, consider the following before you start:

- Do your research into which therapy suits your needs.
- Use word of mouth for possible practitioners.
- Check that they are registered with their regulatory body.
- Talk to several possible practitioners.
- Trust your gut feeling. The patient–practitioner relationship is key to success, so you have to "gel" with the practitioner.
- Give yourself a little time to reflect before making your final choice.
- Set yourself a time-frame (4–6 months, ideally) and review the treatment at the end of that time.
- Continue conventional medicinal treatment, especially if you are over 35.
- Don't commit to a long course of treatment.
- Don't flit from one treatment to another.

find out more: **acupuncture**

There is increasing evidence that acupuncture and electro-acupuncture can have **fertility-boosting effects**, as well as helping certain medical conditions.

I use acupuncture in my clinic, both to help women conceive naturally and to help those who are going through IVF. There has been an increasing number of studies carried out into the benefits of acupuncture, but still more need to be done. One of the biggest obstacles is the absence of a single standard of care, making a full clinical trial not possible as things currently stand. However, many medical doctors are convinced of its benefits and would like to increase its use for a wide variety of ailments.

how does acupuncture work?

There are 365 acupuncture points – or acupoints – located along invisible pathways called meridians (channels of energy). These points are like tiny valves through which the flow of *qi* (see page 133) can be regulated. By inserting fine needles into these acupoints, the body's own healing response is stimulated and its natural balance is restored.

It is important that you find an acupuncturist who specializes in fertility, especially if you are older or have a known fertility problem. He or she may also advise you to change various other aspects of your life, including your lifestyle and diet (see Steps 5 and 6), in order to help the holistic way in which Chinese medicine approaches treatment.

Treatment is given to support a weak organ and restore balance; the acupoints that are used will depend on the client's medical history (both physical and emotional). Certain acupoints are particularly good for fertility, such as the Door of Infants and the Gate of Life. The meridians associated with fertility and reproduction are the kidneys, spleen, and liver.

In order to re-establish balance in a woman's body and to enhance her fertility, I usually give treatment on a weekly basis. I use acupuncture twice weekly on women undergoing IVF treatment.

acupuncture **benefits**

- It increases blood flow to the uterus.
- It helps with endorphin production, which has effects on the pituitary gland and hormone production.
- It regulates hormonal imbalance.
- It has positive effects on gynaecological problems, such as endometriosis and PCOS (see page 18).

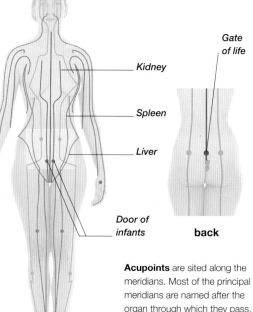

Gate of life
Kidney
Spleen
Liver
Door of infants
back

Acupoints are sited along the meridians. Most of the principal meridians are named after the organ through which they pass. Each organ plays a role in maintaining a smooth flow of *qi*, which in turn allows the body systems to function well.

how is diagnosis made?

A practitioner asks questions about your lifestyle and uses a number of physical checks to diagnose where an imbalance might lie. If you have a fertility problem, he or she will consider the following:

▨ The appearance of your tongue. This is an important diagnostic tool. Each area of your tongue represents a different part of the body. I observe the colour of the tongue and I look for coating and the presence of any cracks.

▨ The sound of your voice.

▨ Your skin tone.

▨ Your body odour.

▨ The warmth of your abdomen relative to the rest of your body. For example, I find that many women with fertility problems have a cold abdomen. Yet, if your *qi* is flowing properly, it should be as warm as the rest of your body. According to the Chinese, the abdomen needs to be warm in order for a baby to grow inside it.

▨ Your pulse. Pulse diagnosis will be made by checking six positions on the wrist, each one relating to specific organs. The quality of your pulse varies throughout your cycle and imbalances can be detected from these changes.

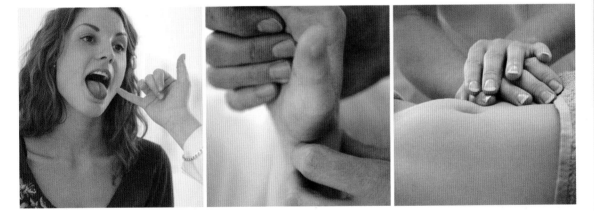

Each area of the tongue represents a different part of the body.

Reading the six distinct pulses forms a crucial part of diagnosis.

Abdominal diagnosis is about temperature, which should be even all over the body.

135

what happens during treatment?

A practitioner will find an acupoint by feeling along the meridian until he or she locates a little dip. A fine needle will be inserted at that point, and the patient may experience a dull sensation, but no pain.

If symptoms suggest a kidney deficiency, for example, acupuncture on specific acupoints along that meridian will support the kidneys and restore balance. According to the Chinese, the kidneys store *jing* or essence. Good *jing* means strong sperm, strong eggs, and healthy children.

The ear is very important in treatment as the Chinese see it as a representation of an inverted fetus, and all the major meridians cross the ear. It has more than 120 acupoints and is especially useful for treating hormonal imbalances.

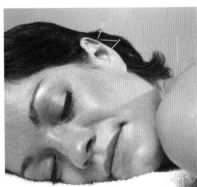

Auricular (ear) acupuncture helps regulate all the body's internal organs, structures and functions.

Q How can osteopathy help fertility?

Osteopathy is a way of detecting and treating malfunctioning parts of the body, such as ligaments, nerves, and joints. In addition, when the body is balanced and working efficiently, it will function with the minimum of wear and tear and leave you with more energy as a result. Osteopaths treat a variety of conditions including postural problems, repetitive strain injuries, and sports injuries. There are three main areas of structural and postural strain:

- the mid-cervical (neck and shoulders)
- the dorso-lumbar junction (the mid-to-lower back)
- the sacro-iliac joint (low back and pelvic area).

Bad posture or injury to any one of these areas, for example, can upset the balance between muscles, joints, ligaments, and nerves, which may cause gynaecological problems.

Q What do osteopaths do?

Osteopaths consider each person as an individual and treat the person as a whole, not just the specific symptom. On your first visit, you will be asked questions about your health, your lifestyle, and diet. You will then be asked to undress to your underwear and the osteopath will assess your posture, mobility, and weight so that a full assessment of your problem can be made and a personal treatment plan devised.

Treatment usually involves a mixture of manipulation, stretching, and massage, and each session lasts about 30 to 40 minutes. You will probably need to have several weekly sessions until the symptoms have disappeared. Some people feel slightly light-headed after treatment, but this feeling usually disappears within a couple of hours at most. However, it is advised that you don't do any heavy weight-bearing exercise for 24 hours after treatment.

Q What is cranial osteopathy?

Cranial osteopathy is a refined and subtle type of osteopathic treatment that encourages the release of stresses and tensions throughout the body, through massage of the bones of the skull. The practitioner can feel subtle, rhythmical shape changes. He then assesses which stresses your body is under and treats them through gentle movements that cause no discomfort. Treatment lengths are similar to those of conventional osteopathy. Cranial osteopathy may help the pituitary gland to function properly if there is a hormonal imbalance that may be affecting fertility. And by rebalancing the body and releasing internal stresses, the treatment can be beneficial for overall health and well-being.

Cranial osteopaths are qualified practitioners who have gone on to specialize in cranial osteopathy, although there is currently no formal recognition of post-graduate training.

Q Is osteopathy regulated?

Osteopathy is one of the few CAMs to be regulated (along with chiropractic techniques). The Statutory Register of the General Osteopathic Council (GOsC) opened in 1998, and since 2000 the title "osteopath" has been protected by law. As a result, it is a criminal offence for people to describe themselves as an osteopath in the UK unless they are registered with the GOsC. Only practitioners meeting the high standards of safety and competence are eligible to join this register, and

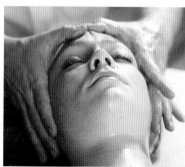

Cranial osteopathy may help the pituitary gland to function properly.

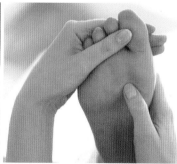

Reflexology is a recognized relaxation therapy, which may boost fertility.

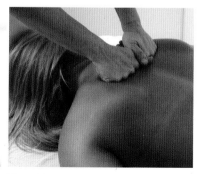

Manual lymphatic drainage uses massage to help the body dispose of waste.

professional indemnity insurance cover is also a requirement. Osteopaths undertake four- to five-year honours degree programmes underpinned by clinical training before they can qualify.

Q Can reflexology help boost fertility?

Reflexology is an ancient complementary medicine involving massaging specific points on the feet (and to a lesser extent, on the hands). Nerve endings are stimulated and this causes changes in other parts of the body. It is not a diagnostic tool but it can detect signs of disorder or disease. It takes a holistic approach, and rather than treating a specific illness, it aims to rebalance the body's systems so that they work in harmony. It cannot cure fertility problems such as blocked fallopian tubes or endometriosis, but research indicates that it could help to improve uterine blood flow and restore regular menstrual cycles among women who suffer from conditions such as PCOS, unexplained infertility, dysmenorrhoea (painful periods), and amenorrhoea (absence of periods – see page 35). More research will be needed to establish whether there is indeed a link but certainly reflexology is a recognized form of relaxation therapy and may help some of these disorders and boost fertility.

Q What is cognitive behaviour therapy (CBT) and can it help with fertility problems?

CBT is a psychological treatment in which cognitive techniques (that challenge negative thoughts) are combined with behavioural techniques (including relaxation techniques or fear reduction techniques) to relieve symptoms of anxiety and depression. As a result, symptoms of stress are reduced or disappear, outlook on life improves, as does general physical and mental health. CBT works on the belief that unwanted thinking patterns and behaviour are learned over a long period of time but can be unlearned using appropriate techniques, exercises, and practice. In 10 to 20 sessions of treatment, you learn to, in effect, reprogramme your way of thinking and reacting to certain events, allowing you to cope with them.

CBT is good for treating an overactive stress response, anxiety and depression, panic attacks, bulimia, ME and chronic fatigue syndrome, post-traumatic stress disorder, and phobias. These conditions can seriously impair well-being and hence have underlying effects on fertility.

Q What's the theory behind manual lymphatic drainage (MLD)?

Developed by the Danish physiotherapist Dr Emil Vodder in the 1930s, MLD, as its name suggests, deals with the lymphatic system, which is part of the body's waste disposal system. This complex network of lymph nodes and ducts, as well as other lymphatic organs, drains a clear fluid called lymph from body tissues and filters it to trap bacteria, toxins, and cell debris before returning it to the bloodstream to maintain the fluid balance in the body. Lymph also contains numerous proteins as well as lymphocytes, which are white blood cells vital for the body's immune system.

Muscle movement is responsible for the flow of lymph around the body and illness or poor health cause the system to become slow or even blocked, which weakens our bodies. All around our body there are lymph nodes that we tend to notice when we are unwell – particularly those in our neck and under our arms – because they often become swollen. Those in the groin filter waste in the lower part of the body, including the pelvic area.

There is no actual drainage involved in manual lymphatic drainage; instead, gentle manual pressure is applied to the skin in slow, rhythmic movements to stimulate the lymphatic vessels and promote the uptake of waste-containing fluid. This helps to unblock the system and restore good lymphatic flow. Each session lasts approximately one hour and it is usually deeply relaxing – as indeed are all forms of massage.

Q Can MLD improve fertility?

Although no studies have been done to show a link between MLD and fertility, I recommend MLD to women who are trying to get pregnant, either naturally or through IVF treatment, or to women who are in between courses of fertility treatment to help get the body's systems back in balance. I believe that a healthy lymphatic system helps to:

- keep the immune system functioning well
- reduce symptoms of painful periods
- improve digestive disorders
- improve sleep.

As MLD can help to improve lymphatic flow, it could improve the chances of a woman getting pregnant.

"If your next step is to try assisted conception you need to do so **as a couple**, so you can support each other through **the highs and lows**"

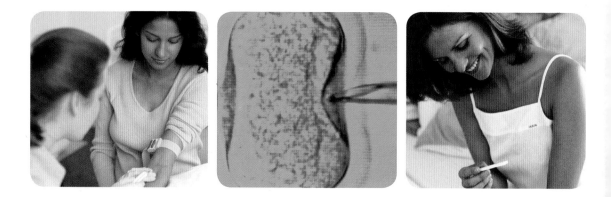

step**nine**
assisted
conception

Your questions answered on:

step 9: **assisted conception**

> If you have **not conceived** and feel you have already tried to **maximize your chances** of getting pregnant naturally, you will have to decide whether or not to try assisted conception. **Various options** are available, ranging from taking drugs to boost ovulation to IVF. This step will help you to understand what the main options involve

Q When should assisted conception be considered?

Each individual and each couple present a unique set of circumstances, but I believe you should seek help with assisted conception only once you feel you have done all you can to get pregnant naturally. Throughout the book I have provided a plan for getting pregnant that includes a health and fertility check for you and your partner, as well as nutritional and lifestyle advice. The aim is to combine these elements in order to maximize your chances of getting pregnant. At this stage, you should go back through the book to see if there are any areas left unchecked. If you think you have ticked all the boxes and gone down every avenue suggested, then you are probably ready to move on.

I feel some younger women are quick to rush down the IVF route before considering whether other treatment options might be more suitable for them initially. Indeed, they may be investigating assisted conception before they have addressed lifestyle and health issues.

If you are under 35, it is perfectly acceptable to consult your GP if nothing has happened after a year of trying, so he or she can arrange for you and your partner to have certain tests done to make sure there is nothing wrong. After that, depending on the test results and how you feel,

you may want to investigate some form of assisted conception. If you are over 35, have been trying to get pregnant for more than six months, and feel you have done all you can, including making appropriate diet and lifestyle changes, I would advise you not to waste any more fertility time, but to seek medical advice now.

Q Who should we consult for advice first of all?

The first thing to do is to see your GP. Some are very good, while others have a more "arms' length" relationship with their patients. Whichever category your GP falls into, make sure you are very clear about what you are hoping to get out of the appointment. You will have only a short length of time with him or her, so have your questions written down so that you don't forget any, be clear in your mind about what you want to come away with (is it a referral to a specialist, and if so, who and where, private or NHS?), otherwise you are going to leave feeling very frustrated. Calculate in advance how long you have been trying for a baby, and do some research beforehand about the different treatment options available so that you are as informed as possible.

If your GP arranges for you to have some tests, make sure you understand exactly what these are for (see pages 142–143). Be assertive (though not aggressive!) and do not accept a GP's recommendation that you should come back in six months if you are still not pregnant, especially if you fall into any of the following categories:

▨ You are over 35.
▨ Your menstrual cycle is irregular.
▨ You have had an ectopic pregnancy in the past.
▨ You have had any miscarriages in the past.

Zita's **tip**

You have a right for your worries to be **taken seriously**, and for investigations to be done.

■ There is a history of premature ovarian failure (early menopause – see page 14) in your family.
■ Your partner has not yet had a sperm test.
■ Your partner has had tests done and the results are not normal.
■ You are becoming emotional and feel increasingly desperate to conceive.

Q Should couples consult together?

I firmly believe that if you are going down the assisted conception route, you need to do so as a couple. It is a journey that is fraught with emotional highs and lows and, if you are not both fully committed, cracks could start to appear in your relationship. It is very important that you are in this together, that you sit down and have a full discussion about how each of you feels, and how far you are prepared to go to have a baby. Some of my clients are very disappointed that they have to go down the IVF route. They feel they have failed and are often very frightened as well because they are wondering if this is their last chance to have a baby. I always tell them that if they are supported, they will be able to go through absolutely anything. The most important thing with IVF, therefore, is to be fully supported by your partner and by anyone else you choose to tell.

I often find that men have only a vague idea, if any, of what the treatment involves and of the actual cost of assisted conception, whereas women, within 24 hours of deciding to seek treatment, have done all the research and have an almost encyclopaedic knowledge of the subject. It can work well if the woman does the research – which she usually wants to do anyway – and then offers a précis to her partner, so that decisions can then be reached jointly, and he never feels left out of the process. It is not that the man is less interested, it is just that the woman is often the one who is most involved in the actual treatment, and therefore the one who is the most committed to researching the information fully.

Q Which tests will we need to have done initially?

A GP can arrange for you to get blood tests done and these will show whether or not you have a healthy hormonal balance and are ovulating consistently (see page 143). Your partner should also have a semen analysis test.

It is vital that you are both investigated at this stage, to avoid the situation where one person is investigated while the other does nothing, only to discover months later that the problem lies with the partner, and valuable time has been lost. Ask whether these tests will be done at a local fertility clinic or at a hospital pathology lab, as the latter, particularly when it comes to semen analysis, may be less accurate and informative than if the test samples are sent to a specialist fertility clinic (see Step 3 for more on semen analysis).

Q What do the blood tests check for?

Simple blood (serum) tests are carried out to check for any hormonal imbalance that may be affecting your fertility. If you are just starting out, these tests will be done by your GP, or if you are at a fertility clinic, they will be done there.

The first test is done on days 1 to 3 of your cycle and measures your FSH level. This hormone stimulates the growth and development of ovarian follicles and the level of FSH gives an indication of the quality of your eggs and

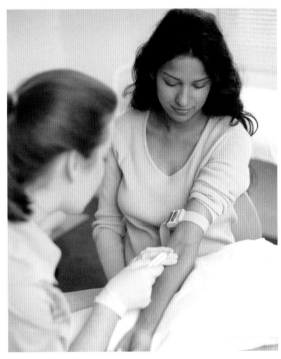

Blood tests carried out as a first line of investigation will help establish whether or not you have a healthy hormonal balance.

your ovarian reserve. Women who are approaching the menopause (perimenopausal) or who are menopausal have high FSH levels and do not respond well to IVF. Raised FSH levels cause much concern for many of the women I see.

The levels of other hormones, including oestradiol and LH, will also be measured. Raised levels of luteinizing hormone (LH) may indicate polycystic ovary syndrome (see page 22), and increased levels of prolactin may indicate problems with ovulation. Some clinics now also use a newer test, called the anti-mullerian hormone (AMH) test (see page 12), which appears to be a more accurate marker of ovarian reserve.

A second blood test is done on day 21 (of a 28-day cycle, or on the appropriate day if the cycle is shorter or longer). It measures the level of progesterone and shows whether or not ovulation has taken place. The test needs to be done about a week after ovulation, and therefore about a week before your next period is due. However, it is not easy to work out the exact date, so ideally you should time the test for about a week after your peak day of fertility (the last day of the clearer, wetter, slippery secretions – see page 40).

Hopefully, your period will start about seven days after the test. Don't panic, though, if the test comes back saying you have not ovulated: it may be due to the fact that the test was not done on the right day after all, or that you simply did not ovulate during that cycle (women do not necessarily ovulate on every cycle). Only if the test repeatedly comes back with a low progesterone level would this alert you to a problem.

Further tests might be done if you have a history of recurrent miscarriage. Increasingly, experts have come to realize that some women have blood-clotting disorders that may be the cause of miscarriage. In some cases, drugs such as aspirin, heparin, or steroids may be used to improve the chances of maintaining a pregnancy. This is a highly controversial area but specialist fertility clinics and miscarriage clinics can now help many women.

Q My FSH levels are high: what effect does that have?

FSH is released by the pituitary gland and its function is to stimulate the growth and maturation of the egg follicles. If levels are raised, this means your body is having to try harder to ripen the egg, and the reason for that is likely to be that your eggs are of poor quality and that your ovarian reserve is low. As IVF relies on egg stimulation and collection, it follows that the lower your FSH level the better your chances.

▥ Levels below 6 (pg/ml) are very encouraging for women hoping to undergo IVF treatment.

▥ Anything below 10 is also considered acceptable for starting IVF.

▥ Levels of 11–13 indicate a higher than normal level of FSH, suggesting that the ovaries are not responding well to stimulation by FSH; IVF may not be possible unless levels fall.

▥ Levels of 14–17 will give little response, and suggest very poor egg quality.

▥ Levels of 17 and above mean you are unlikely to respond to egg stimulation.

You should remember, however, that though a poor (high) reading indicates poor egg quality and ovarian reserve, women (especially those over 40) with low FSH levels can also have poor-quality eggs.

lowering **FSH levels**

High levels of FSH are not good news, as your hopes of starting IVF may be dashed. Try some of the tips below to see if you can lower FSH levels. Be aware, however, that once high, even if they come down, the outcome is not always good, especially if you are older.

▥ Try acupuncture.

▥ Reduce your stress levels (see page 84).

▥ Avoid coffee and tea.

▥ Take gentle exercise (and lose weight if you need to).

▥ Eat foods that are good sources of phyto-oestrogens, such as pulses, oats, broccoli, and linseeds (see Steps 5, 6, and 8).

▥ Take supplements of zinc and vitamin B-complex and essential fatty acids such as omega-3.

Q I have been told I need to go for further tests. What might these involve?

If the results of your blood tests have shown that your hormone levels (and hence ovulation) are normal, then the next step is to see if there are any blockages in your fallopian tubes that might be preventing the progress of the egg or sperm, or if there are uterine problems that are impeding implantation. You will be referred to a hospital for these tests and they will usually be carried out in the first half of your menstrual cycle.

Q I have to have a hysterosalpingogram (HSG). What is that?

This may sound scary but is in fact a routine test. It involves a small tube being inserted into the cervix and liquid dye being squirted through it. Using radiographs, the reproductive organs can then be visualized to see if there are any blockages, obstructions, or abnormalities, particularly in the fallopian tubes. Sometimes the procedure can cause cramping or discomfort, although the level of pain is variable.

---

find out more: **further investigations**

If there is a blockage in your fallopian tubes, a laparoscopy and/or a hysteroscopy (see below) may be done to check the extent of the obstruction and to look at the uterine cavity. The severity of the blockage will determine the best course of action and IVF treatment may be recommended.

If you have fibroids (see page 23), your specialist can use these tests to help determine their size and number and to assess whether they are likely to be affecting your fertility. After treatment, you may be able to return to trying to get pregnant naturally. If endometriosis (see page 22) is detected, again treatment may enable you to return to planning a natural conception.

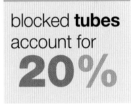

blocked **tubes** account for

20%

of female infertility.

Laparoscopy is used to look for disorders of the reproductive organs. This is done under general anaesthetic. A laparoscope, a rigid instrument resembling a small telescope, and an instrument to manipulate the internal organs are inserted through small incisions in the abdomen. Gas is pumped through the laparoscope so the organs can separate and be seen clearly. A second instrument may also be inserted through the vagina.

Hysteroscopy is used to see inside the uterus and fallopian tubes. It reveals abnormalities such as fibroids or adhesions. This procedure is done under mild sedation or local anaesthetic, or under general anaesthetic at the same time as a laparoscopy. A hysteroscope, which is a small viewing instrument, is inserted through the vagina, and the uterus and the fallopian tubes are filled with gas to allow them to be seen clearly. Light provides a clear view.

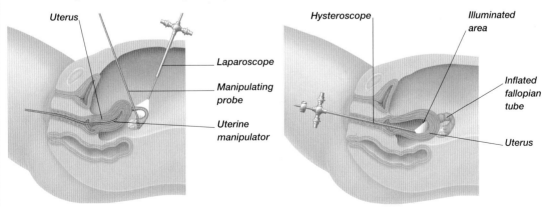

Uterus
Laparoscope
Manipulating probe
Uterine manipulator

Hysteroscope
Illuminated area
Inflated fallopian tube
Uterus

Q Do we need private treatment or can we get help on the NHS?

It saddens me to say this but the reality is that, in the NHS system, the waiting times for any further investigations (and this is irrespective of whether you decide to pursue IVF) can vary from area to area and may be as long as six to nine months. You may well not wish to wait that long. A private consultation with a gynaecologist, rather than seeing your GP as a first port of call, possibly followed by having the intial tests done privately, can save you a lot of time.

It can work out that, if you find something is wrong with you or your partner, you can go straight back into the NHS for treatment, armed with the results of the tests, which can often be the most time-consuming part of seeking help. And if you are then going on to try IVF treatment on the NHS, you will also have saved time by getting the tests done while you are on the NHS waiting list for your treatment.

Ten questions to ask a clinic

There are many questions that you may want to ask at an initial consultation, but the list below (see also the HFEA website, pages 184–185) may be helpful:

- Why have you recommended this particular treatment to me?
- Are there alternative treatments? If so, why are they less suitable for me?
- Which drugs will I have to take and what are their common side effects?
- Can you break down the costs for me, so that I am clear about all the financial implications of the treatment?
- Could there be further costs at a later stage?
- What are the next steps – what tests need to be done?
- When can I expect treatment to begin?
- How many people in my/our situation have you treated in the last two years and how many have had a baby? What are your overall statistics?
- What kind of counselling/support do you provide?
- If this treatment doesn't work, do I have any other options?

Q What happens once the results from the preliminary tests are back?

If your tests reveal there are problems, your GP will refer you to a specialist at a fertility clinic who will be responsible for your ongoing treatment. Depending on the results, you may then be referred to a gynaecologist who is a specialist in reproductive medicine (and therefore trained in dealing with men and women together), a urologist (if the man has urological or erectile/ejaculatory problems), or a clinical andrologist (who specializes in all problems related to men's reproduction). Tests will then be done to investigate any problems further and to determine which form of fertility treatment might be most suitable for you as a couple.

Q What should we look for when choosing a clinic?

The Human Fertilization and Embryology Authority (HFEA) website (see Resources, pages 184–185) gives detailed advice and information, including how to choose a fertility clinic, how to understand the clinics' success rates, and which questions you should ask when you visit a clinic. Here are a few of my own suggestions as to what to look out for when choosing a fertility clinic.

- If you are aged 40+, choose a clinic that has proven experience and a good success rate in this age category. Age is an important factor, as success rates for assisted conception decline as you get older. Ask any clinic you visit what their success rate has been in your age category during the last two years.

- Depending on your health history, bear in mind that some clinics have exclusion policies (which may relate to age, FSH levels, marital status, sexuality, and HIV and hepatitis C infection). Ask them about this before making an appointment to see them.

- Ask what treatments and services are offered. The most common complaint I get about some clinics is that they offer poor patient care and support, and yet emotional support and preparation for treatment is vital. However, many clinics do have counsellors on site.

- In my experience, clinics that tailor-make the treatment to each couple rather than following a standard "one-size-fits-all" protocol appear to have a better success rate. Enquire what the situation is with any prospective clinic.

- Don't let yourself be rushed or intimidated during a consultation, and make sure you come away with a clear understanding of what has been said.
- Don't be frightened of asking awkward questions, and ask again if you don't understand the answers.
- Consider paying for an initial consultation at more than one clinic to ensure you find one you are comfortable with.
- If you are on your third or fourth treatment, ask your consultant what aspect of your care he or she plans to change for any subsequent cycles.
- After any failed cycle, make sure you can have a follow-up consultation to discuss all aspects of your treatment.

Q Do clinics often get booked up in advance?

Whether you are an NHS or a private patient, you should always assume that you will have to wait for your first appointment at a fertility clinic. Plan ahead because some consultants have long waiting lists, even in the private sector. And remember, too, that if you decide to have IVF, you may not be able to start straight after your initial appointment because there may be other tests you have to undergo.

Q What questions should we ask at the first clinic appointment?

You need to be fully prepared when you go to your first consultation at the clinic you have chosen. Take your time with the consultant – remember, you are the client who is paying for his or her advice, and you have a right to ask any questions that you want and to get clear answers to them. Get a rough idea of the time element: when tests will be done, when treatment would start, when future appointments might be, so that you can plan ahead accordingly. And make sure all costs are broken down for you so that you are not taken by surprise by an unexpected bill half way through the treatment.

If you have doubts about the clinic after your first appointment, consider going to see a second one, if only to put your mind at rest. It is vital that you are entirely happy with the clinic and comfortable with the staff who will be looking after you because you need to have the utmost faith in the team and in the treatment they are proposing. At the end of the initial appointment, you need to come away feeling really positive, and knowing exactly what you will be doing and why.

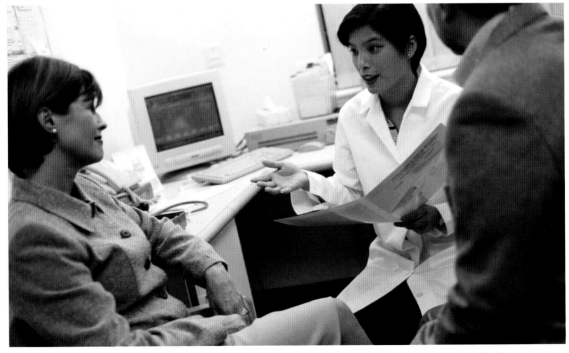

Once preliminary tests are under way with your GP, you will be referred to a fertility clinic to discuss your treatment choices.

Q What are the main treatment options for assisted conception?

Following your test results it may be recommended that you go down the route of assisted conception. These techniques include:

- ovulation induction (OI)
- intrauterine insemination (IUI)
- in vitro fertilization (IVF) and intra-cytoplasmic sperm injection (ICSI).

It may be that you could start with the less invasive form of treatment, OI, and postpone trying the more invasive options until later. Alternatively, there may be only one treatment suitable for your particular situation. This will depend on your age, the outcome of tests both you and your partner will have undergone, discussions with your clinician, and discussions with your partner.

Q What is ovulation induction (OI)?

This is also called ovarian stimulation and it involves taking a drug called clomiphene citrate (the brand name is Clomid or Serophene) in tablet form. This stimulates the production of various hormones that are responsible for ovulation. Regular ultrasound scanning of the ovaries during the cycle is essential to ensure that not too many eggs are produced, which could lead to ovarian

hyperstimulation syndrome (see opposite page). Because of the associated risks of long-term use, clomiphene should not be given for more than three months at a time. It can be given for a total of six months, but there should be a one-month break after the first three months. Other drugs, given as injections or tablets, are also prescribed for ovarian stimulation but clomiphene is used most commonly.

Q How does OI work?

Clomiphene is taken from day 2 to day 5 of your cycle. The drug binds to oestrogen receptor sites in the brain, making the body think that oestrogen secretion is too low. This causes the hypothalamus to produce more GnRH (gonadotrophin-releasing hormone). GnRH tells the pituitary gland to release more LH and FSH. This results in an egg starting to mature in a follicle, ready for ovulation. HCG (human chorionic gonadotrophin) injections may also be given to boost final maturation of follicles. HCG is usually given 36 to 40 hours before sexual intercourse or IUI (see opposite) takes place.

Q Who is OI suitable for?

Women whose periods are irregular, as a result of a diagnosed hormonal imbalance, and those who are under the age of 35, are most likely to benefit. OI can help women

pros and cons of ovulation induction	
pros	**cons**
Not invasive, although sometimes an injection of the hormone hCG (human chorionic gonadotrophin) is given to provide a final boost to a follicle and enable it to mature and release its egg.	You may be wasting valuable fertility time if age is not on your side.
It is cheap in cost compared to IVF and ICSI.	Side effects can include nausea, headaches, weight gain, bloating and, for higher doses, hot flushes and breast tenderness.
For suitable women, the chances of success are good.	15 per cent of women go on to develop ovarian hyperstimulation, where too many eggs are produced (see opposite page). This can also increase the risk of multiple births.
Worth a try for a few months (not a long-term option).	There may be serious side effects for some women; talk to your doctor about any family history of gynaecological cancers and any other concerns.

with polycystic ovary syndrome (see page 22), those whose production of LH is faulty and prevents the ovarian follicles from maturing properly, or those who are producing insufficient amounts of progesterone after ovulation in the luteal phase (a luteal phase defect – see page 38), which inhibits the implantation of a fertilized egg in the womb.

Q What is the success rate of OI?

Although the success of OI varies according to each individual's circumstances, 80 per cent of women with irregular or no periods will ovulate as a result of the treatment and 50 per cent will conceive during the three-month course of treatment. The majority of pregnancies occur within the first three months; very few occur after six months of treatment. It also appears to be the case that the longer you are on the drug, then the lower your chances of conception. Women over 40 usually have poor results.

Q What is ovarian hyperstimulation syndrome (OHSS)?

In about 15 per cent of women who are treated with OI or IVF, too many eggs are produced; this is called OHSS. This is why women following IVF treatment (and to a lesser extent OI) need to be monitored closely and have regular ultrasound scans to check the number and development of follicles in each ovary. If many follicles develop in an ovary, doctors will suspend treatment and the woman will be told to rest and to drink plenty of water (at least 2 litres a day). Occasionally, the abdomen and thorax become engorged with fluid, and in very rare cases OHSS can lead to thrombosis, heart attack, or stroke. Symptoms to watch out for include:

- nausea and vomiting
- severe abdominal pain
- difficulty breathing
- feeling faint.

Q What is intrauterine insemination (IUI)?

IUI is a procedure in which good-quality active sperm are placed directly into the uterus – and therefore close to an egg. This is done around the time of ovulation, which is determined either by an ultrasound scan or using an ovulation predictor kit. IUI gives the sperm a helping hand by enabling them to avoid the first hurdle: having to make their way through the cervical mucus and into the uterus. Natural fertilization still takes place in the fallopian tubes. With IUI alone, there is a 6 to 8 per cent rate of conception per cycle. Used in conjunction with clomiphene, this goes up to 10 to 12 per cent.

pros and cons of IUI	
pros	**cons**
IUI on its own is not particularly invasive and may not necessarily require hormonal treatment.	You may need daily injections of certain fertility drugs.
The procedure itself is quick and causes little/no pain.	The success rate of IUI on its own is low. Even if used in conjunction with fertility drugs the chances of conception are not very high.
Although it is not a long-term option, it may be worth trying before moving on to more complex fertility treatment such as IVF.	Some couples say they feel "in limbo" at their clinic and suffer from having less attention than couples who are undergoing full IVF; they sometimes feel they are not getting enough physical or emotional support.
	Undergoing this treatment could be wasting fertility time: three cycles of IUI could delay you by up to six months.

Zita's tip
Research is key. Find out all the **facts and figures** about your clinic before starting IVF.

Q What does the IUI procedure involve?

Your partner will have to provide a sperm sample, which will be washed and sorted to make sure that only the healthiest sperm are used. These are then placed into the uterus using a catheter that has been inserted via the cervix. Treatment takes only a few minutes and generally causes little or no pain. A few women experience some cramping afterwards. You will be advised to lie down for 30 minutes after treatment, and to rest for a while thereafter.

IUI takes place as close to ovulation as possible. Some clinics schedule two treatments, one just before ovulation and the other during ovulation. Ask your clinic which protocol (method of treatment) it follows. To predict ovulation accurately, you will have ultrasound scans at regular intervals, and you will also have to use a home ovulation kit to detect the surge of luteinizing hormone (LH) that occurs around ovulation.

IUI is often carried out alongside ovulation induction treatment, including an hCG injection (see page 146). If this is the case, it is not a form of treatment that can be used repeatedly.

Q Who is IUI suitable for?

There are a number of situations where IUI might be considered. These include the following:
- when the woman is aged 35 or under
- when a woman has been using OI drugs but the treatment on its own has been unsuccessful
- for women whose fallopian tubes are not blocked
- where there is unexplained infertility
- where there is no problem with sperm quality and the sperm count is OK, ie, there are a minimum 1 million washed sperm per millilitre.
- for artificial insemination via donor sperm
- for gay couples.

Q What is in vitro fertilization (IVF)?

This is now the best-known form of assisted conception and the one that many people immediately think of when faced with the possibility of treatment. It is a complex procedure and should not be undertaken lightly. IVF involves retrieving multiple mature eggs just before ovulation and fertilizing them in a Petri dish (hence the "in glass" meaning of *in vitro*) in laboratory conditions. The resulting embryos (if there are more than one) are then graded and the best – though a maximum of two – are then transferred, via a catheter inserted through the cervix, to the uterus, where it is hoped they will implant.

Clinics are now aiming to do a single embryo transfer wherever possible as research has shown that replacing a single embryo, rather than two, does not change the overall pregnancy rate, and almost halves the twin pregnancy rate. As singleton pregnancies are much safer for both mother and baby, many clinics now believe that a good-quality single embryo is preferable for a successful outcome to IVF.

Q Who is IVF suitable for?

IVF is not suitable for everyone but it may be the only way in which some women can get pregnant. For example, it can help:
- women whose fallopian tubes have become blocked.
- women with a hormonal imbalance who have not responded to other forms of treatment.
- couples with unexplained infertility.
- men with low sperm counts or poor-quality sperm (see ICSI on page 155).
- couples who carry the gene for certain specific genetic disorders such as cystic fibrosis. These couples can now undergo a procedure called pre-implantation diagnosis (PGD) in which embryos are tested and only those that are free from the disorder are transferred.
- couples who require a donor egg to become pregnant, either because the woman is no longer producing eggs (perhaps as a result of a previous illness) or because her eggs are not able to mature properly. See page 151 for more on the issues surrounding donor eggs and sperm.

Women who are over 35 can and regularly do get pregnant using IVF. As ever, though, the younger the woman is, the better are her chances of going on to have a successful pregnancy.

Q What is the success rate of IVF?

This varies considerably and depends on many factors, including the clinic, the type of patient it treats, and maternal age. The rate can be approaching 50 per cent in a few clinics or as little as 10 per cent in others.

The average success rate per treatment cycle in the UK for IVF using fresh eggs is:
- 28.2 per cent for women under 35
- 23.6 per cent for women aged 35–37
- 18.3 per cent for women aged 38–39
- 10.6 per cent for women aged 40–42
- 3 per cent for women aged 43–44
- 1 per cent or less for women aged 45 and over.

Remember that some clinics do have much higher success rates than these averages.

Q If IVF is the best option, what happens next?

The first thing to do if you have opted for IVF treatment is to find a clinic that you think will give you the best chance of success, given your particular situation. Bear in mind that clinics have different age cut-off points, or different exclusion policies regarding potential patients (see pages 144–145). The HFEA website (see Resources, pages 184-184) gives information about choosing a clinic and how to interpret the often confusing statistics which are produced by individual clinics. Many clinics have a success rate approaching 50 per cent for women under the age of 35, and even for those over 35, their figures may be encouraging. This may mean, though, that they refuse to treat older women, or those who have particular fertility or health problems.

Be sure to also consider other factors such as the clinic's location, waiting times for treatment, and cost (including for all drugs and tests). Learn to be savvy about what the information really means, and don't be frightened to ask awkward questions.

Q Can I get help with funding?

Government guidelines say women aged between 23 and 39 are able to have one IVF cycle free on the NHS. However, each Primary Care Trust (PCT) decides what the eligibility criteria should be, and this can therefore vary from one region to another. You can contact your PCT direct to find out what the situation is in your area, but be warned that waiting lists for treatment are invariably long, and funding, if there is any, is scarce.

Q How much time should be allowed for the various treatment options?

It is very important to take time into account when calculating which options to try. OI takes three months, for example, IUI another three, then IUI with clomiphene another three. That is already a total of nine months, not allowing for any breaks. IVF takes place over one menstrual cycle – but you should try not to cram in as many cycles as possible into a year. Plan ahead, because no matter which treatment you use, the months will add up.

pros and cons of IVF

pros	cons
IVF has increasingly good success rates, depending on individual circumstances and clinics.	It is very expensive. Costs run into thousands of pounds per treatment cycle and, although about 25 per cent of IVF cycles in the UK are now funded by the NHS, this figure varies considerably from one health authority to another.
It is the most thorough form of assisted conception.	
It is the only chance of conceiving for some couples.	It is very time consuming.
	IVF is emotionally and physically demanding.
	There is a high risk of multiple births and all the associated health problems for mother and babies.

Q What are IVF protocols?

IVF protocols refer to the sequence of procedures that take place in order to retrieve eggs ready for fertilization. There are two main protocols – the long and the short protocol – and which one you will be on will depend on your clinic and on the results of the tests you have already undergone.

The long protocol is for women who have normal hormone levels and regular cycles. The short protocol is for women with high FSH levels, or who have previously responded poorly to ovarian stimulation.

the **shorter protocol**

This shorter protocol does not involve a period of down-regulation, as in the long protocol (see below).

- A suppression drug is given on day 2 of the cycle to prevent maturation and ovulation.
- There is no down-regulation period.
- Instead, FSH injections begin on day 3.
- Thereafter, the short and long protocols work in the same way (see below).

long protocol stages

	down-regulation	manipulation	maturation	egg retrieval
what is it?	Your natural production of FSH, which normally starts to rise on days 2–3 of your cycle, is suppressed, or "down-regulated", with drugs administered either by nasal spray or by injection. The follicles that would have ripened for this cycle are not now able to mature.	Your next reproductive cycle can now be manipulated by FSH injections (sometimes combined with LH as well). These stimulate more than the usual one follicle (in a normal cycle) to mature.	An injection of human chorionic gonadotrophin (HCG) is given to help final maturation.	On average, 8–12 eggs are collected from the 10–20 follicles that had begun to ripen at the start of the manipulated cycle.
when does it happen?	Suppression drugs are administered starting on day 21 of the preceding cycle, and are usually given for 7 days. Your period starts 7–9 days afterwards.	FSH injections start on day 3–5 of your next cycle.	The injection is given around days 9-10, but this will vary according to your ultrasound scans.	36 hours later the eggs are retrieved, just before ovulation. They are fertilized *in vitro* following the procedure described on pages 152–153.
tests and scans	Blood tests will be done to check your levels of hormones at the start of your cycle.	Ultrasound scans may be carried out to check for any problems, and further blood tests may be done.	You will have scans to check development of the follicles and blood tests to check hormone levels.	

step nine

150

assisted conception

Make sure you have a personal **contact at your clinic** who will respond to variations in your cycle.

Q What is natural IVF?

A few clinics offer this treatment, which does not involve ovary-stimulating drugs. The fully ripe egg is retrieved just before ovulation and mixed with sperm and, if an embryo develops, it will be implanted into the uterus a few days later. A ten per cent success rate per treatment cycle means that it is less reliable than conventional IVF, although over three or four attempts, pregnancy rates are similar. This method suits some couples – and costs far less than standard IVF – but given that the process is still time consuming and emotionally draining, many prefer to stick to the normal drug-assisted version of treatment.

Q What is in vitro maturation (IVM)?

This is a new and exciting development in IVF. Here, immature eggs are collected from the ovary and ripened outside the woman's body. They are then fertilized using traditional IVF. It is suitable for women whose eggs cannot mature naturally, or who are at risk of ovarian hyperstimulation (especially those with PCOS – see page 22), or who are about to undergo cancer treatment (their immature eggs can be frozen). IVM costs much less than standard IVF because fewer expensive drugs are used before the eggs can be collected, reducing the overall cost. This experimental but promising technique has shown encouraging results (up to 30 per cent success rate with suitable women) in the few clinics worldwide that offer it.

Q What happens if we need donor eggs or sperm?

Donor eggs or sperm are used if conception is unlikely to occur using either a woman's eggs or her partner's sperm. Donor sperm is also used for women who want to conceive but do not have a male partner.

If you are receiving donated sperm, your cycle will be monitored using either an ovulation predictor kit or ultrasound scanning. You may be given fertility drugs to ensure ovulation. At ovulation, sperm are placed directly in the vagina, cervix, or uterus using artificial insemination. IVF will be used if this method is not successful after a few attempts.

Donor sperm was the only treatment option for some male fertility problems until the technique of ICSI was developed (see page 155), but now the use of donor sperm is less common. Donor eggs are increasingly required as more and more older women are seeking assisted conception. Egg donation is physically demanding for the donor, as she has to go through an IVF protocol right up to and including the egg collection stage. The recipient's own cycle will have been manipulated to match the donor's, so that embryo transfer (assuming the man's sperm fertilizes at least one egg) can take place, as it would with a standard IVF treatment cycle. If transfer needs to be delayed, the embryos are frozen and transferred at a suitable time. Egg donation tends to produce better results than standard IVF because the eggs are all taken from women under 35. What is more, the recipient has not had to take the ovulation-stimulation drugs, leaving her endometrium (uterine lining) in a more natural state.

Since April 2005, people donating sperm, eggs, or embryos in the UK no longer have the right to remain anonymous. Around 800 children are born every year in the UK as a result of sperm or egg donation, and although these children will have no financial or legal claims on their genetic parent, they will, from the age of 18, be able to contact the Human Fertilization and Embryology Authority to obtain details of who their genetic mother or father is. Surprisingly, since the change in the law, numbers of newly registered sperm donors have actually risen slightly, although figures for egg donation continue to be very low, leading to long waiting times before treatment can even begin.

If you are considering conceiving using donated gametes (as sperm and eggs are called) you must by law receive counselling to talk through all the complex legal, financial, emotional, and ethical issues involved. Because of the new law, for example, you will probably not be able to keep your decision private, as you might have chosen to do in the past, so you need to reflect on whether you are happy for all to know that your child is only partially genetically related to you. It is also essential that both you and your partner are fully comfortable with any decision you take.

find out more: **IVF procedure**

The build-up to the start of IVF treatment can be nerve-wracking. You may feel that you are facing an obstacle course of tests, scans, and treatments.

It is natural to feel apprehensive at the prospect of IVF, but you will probably find that the procedure is not as bad as you anticipated. For many women, the hardest part of IVF is not the treatment itself but the two weeks that follow while they wait to find out if they are pregnant. Women often also worry about the chances of a multiple pregnancy – but clinics now restrict the number of embryos implanted to one or two.

one study showed a

42%

increase in the success rate of IVF when acupuncture was used.

the procedure

Egg retrieval This is usually carried out under heavy sedation or under general anaesthetic. An ultrasound scan is used to determine the time of ovulation and the eggs are removed from the follicles using a needle and syringe. This is generally done using a vaginal ultrasound probe to guide the needle. The eggs are examined under a microscope and graded. Depending on the clinic, that evening you may start on a course of progesterone, given by injection or as suppositories, to help prepare the uterine lining for an embryo to implant.

Sperm collection At this stage your partner will be required to produce a sperm sample. The sperm will be specially prepared and then placed in a test tube or Petri dish together with the selected eggs (in a special culture medium). These are then incubated.

Fertilization The eggs and sperm will then be examined under a microscope. If fertilization has taken place, two nuclei (one from the egg, one from the sperm) will be visible. Within 48 hours, cell division is well under way, which means the embryos are ready for transferral. Any good-quality embryos that are not used can be frozen for up to five years, in case they are needed for future IVF attempts, although the success rate from using frozen embryos is not as high as with fresh ones.

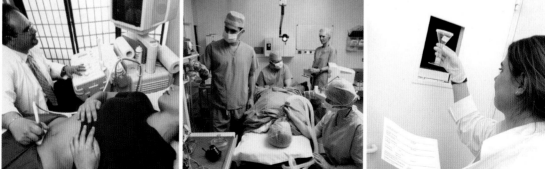

An ultrasound scan helps determine when the eggs are mature enough for retrieval.

Multiple eggs are harvested from the follicles in the ovaries and graded.

Sperm produced by your partner will now be prepared.

what to do while you wait

Once the IVF procedures are complete, you will have to wait two weeks to find out if treatment has been successful. To spend the time well, follow these tips.

- Rest is particularly important for the first three days. After this, continue to take things easy for the remainder of the two weeks.
- Do no exercise other than gentle walking – avoid lifting and anaerobic exercise.
- Relaxation and deep breathing exercises are important.
- Drink 2 litres of water a day (and no coffee or tea).
- Eat healthily and take a good multi-vitamin and mineral supplement including omega-3.
- Visualize the embryo embedding in your uterus, and practise breathing and relaxation exercises.
- Keep yourself occupied so you don't spend all day wondering and worrying.
- Consider acupuncture (with a practitioner experienced in treating IVF patients) as it is thought to make the endometrium more receptive to implantation.
- Don't become obsessed with watching for "symptoms" of pregnancy. The extra progesterone you will be taking can produce confusing side effects.

Drink plenty of water rather than drinks containing caffeine, which can affect fertility.

Embryo transfer The embryos are graded 1 to 4, with grade 1 being the best. Embryos with a high grade seem to produce higher pregnancy rates, but this is by no means always the case. Usually, just one or two suitable embryos are transferred. (Clinics must abide by the guidelines of the Human Fertilization and Embryology Authority, which are intended to prevent multiple births.)

Transfer takes place between 48 hours and five days after fertilization. This is done using a tiny, flexible catheter inserted through the cervix. Embryos are deposited near the top of the uterus. Ideally, you should have an empty bladder so avoid drinking too many fluids on the day of the transfer.

If you were not started on a course of progesterone at the egg retrieval stage, you will be given the hormone now.

The two-week wait This can seem interminable and emotionally draining as patients anxiously count the days to find out if they are pregnant. Rest and recuperation are essential, at least for the first three days after transfer, to give the embryos the best chance to embed in the womb lining. Your clinic will arrange for a blood test to be done after 14 days. This is the only accurate way of knowing if you are pregnant, so if at all possible, try to avoid doing a home pregnancy test beforehand. They can sometimes give misleading results, especially if they are done too early.

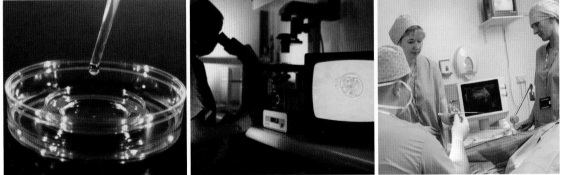

The eggs and sperm are then mixed together in a Petri dish.

The mixture is then examined to see if fertilization has taken place.

Selected embryos will be transferred into the uterus using a small, flexible catheter.

Q I am 41 years old. What are my chances of success with IVF?

Success rates of IVF treatment are good at some clinics, but there is no doubt that they decline sharply with women aged 40 and over. Yet, the number of women over 40 being treated for infertility has nearly doubled since 2000, and one in seven cycles of IVF is performed on women aged between 40 and 45. This is due to several factors, the most common being that couples are waiting longer to start a family, and others are in new relationships and are trying for a second family. As a result, the average age of IVF patients has also increased to nearly 35 years of age.

However, since 1990 there has been little improvement in success rates for women aged over 42, according to the HFEA, and figures for those aged 40 show that live birth rates are nearly half those for women aged just two years younger. This is simply down to biology and the fact that a woman's eggs are as old as she is. Although many women in their forties look and feel younger than ever, and are often in excellent health, this doesn't mean that their eggs are going to be younger than their biological age.

I have to confess that when a woman comes to me at 45 and says that she is having IVF, I am always rather despondent, even though I realize that statistics are only figures. Of course, the woman in question could be included in the one per cent who are successful in getting a healthy baby at the end of their treatment. But I always advise women – and this is vital if you are over 40 – to ask any clinic they are thinking of using "How many people coming through your clinic are successful at my age?" I think you will find that, for women aged 45, the answer is likely to be zero. And if you are over 40, do your research very thoroughly about which clinic can help you best (see pages 144–145 and the HFEA website – pages 184–185 – for a regional breakdown of clinic success rates).

It is also important to bear in mind that there are increased risks associated with older pregnancies. These include a greater risk of miscarriage, ectopic pregnancy, and premature birth. There is also an increased risk of birth defects such as Down's syndrome and of pregnancy complications such as pre-eclampsia.

However, the fact still remains that despite statistics and the way that older women are often given a hard time for wanting to conceive, I am an optimist and am pleased to have helped many women over the age of 40 to get pregnant with IVF.

Q My partner has a low sperm count. Can ICSI help us to conceive?

Intra-cytoplasmic sperm injection (ICSI) is a type of IVF that carries a high fertilization rate and a high live birth rate. The procedure is particularly successful in overcoming male infertility issues arising from problems with sperm, as only a single healthy sperm needs to be isolated and then injected directly into an egg (see opposite page).

ICSI is not an infallible technique: the egg may not be successfully fertilized because it is too immature, too ripe, or of poor quality generally; the sperm that fertilizes the egg may be defective; and not all eggs that are fertilized will go on to divide. However, the success rate of fertilization with ICSI is high.

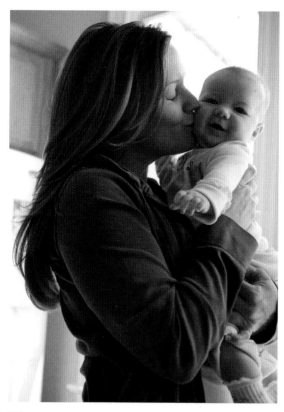

IVF success rates in women aged 40 and over are low yet many women in this age group do have healthy babies with this technique.

find out more: **ICSI**

This is an IVF technique where an individual sperm is isolated and, using a fine glass pipette under a microscope, is injected directly into the centre of an egg that has been harvested using ovarian stimulation and retrieval. The fertilized egg develops into an embryo, which is then cultured, graded, and transferred using the same procedure as in standard IVF (see pages 152–153).

For the woman there is no difference between IVF and ICSI as her IVF protocol and procedures will be the same. The only difference is in how the eggs are fertilized in the laboratory. Sometimes the embryologist will fertilize half the eggs using the standard IVF technique and the other half by ICSI. There is always a dialogue on how to proceed between yourself and the embryologist.

success rate **of ICSI**

- On average, between 60 and 70 per cent of eggs will be fertilized.
- The live birth rates are approximately the same as for standard IVF (an average of 21.6 per cent per treatment cycle).

when is this technique used?

ICSI will be considered when:
- a man's sperm count is very low.
- the sperm are abnormal or have poor motility.
- there is a blockage in the tubes carrying sperm from the testes to the penis.
- previous IVF attempts have failed.
- it is difficult for the eggs to be fertilized using standard IVF.

ICSI can be used as long as a man can produce a single sperm. Even if no sperm are present in the ejaculate, or if, because of illness or injury, there is no ejaculate (for example, following a spinal cord injury), it is possible to retrieve sperm directly from the testes or the tubes leading from the testes. A sperm does not need to be mature or motile, because it is injected directly into the egg.

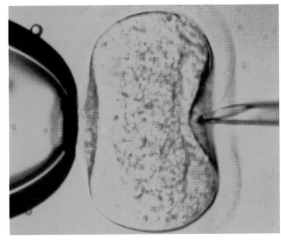

A single sperm is injected into an egg using a fine glass pipette.

pros and cons of ICSI

pros	cons
Similar to those of IVF.	Similar to those of IVF.
The most successful form of fertility treatment for men, accounting for 44 per cent of IVF treatment cycles.	The woman still has to undergo the IVF procedure. The woman's age and reproductive health are still key factors in the success rate of ICSI.

Q How can I **prepare for IVF**?

There are many hurdles to overcome with IVF, and although science can – and does – regularly perform miracles, I always emphasize to my clients that before embarking on treatment there is a lot that you and your partner can do to improve your chances of success. Before starting IVF, it is worth both partners devoting the time to preparing themselves physically, psychologically, and practically to give themselves the best chance of a successful outcome.

Make sure you have ticked all the boxes Go through this book, making sure you have done all you can to maximize your chances of conceiving naturally. Once you feel you have done what you can, or if you think something may be wrong anyway, move on to trying fertility treatment.

Communicate with your partner at all times You are in this together, so make sure you are on the same wavelength from the start. Keep your partner in touch with any research you might be doing.

See your GP Do your research beforehand and go prepared with a list of questions. Be clear about what you want to get out of the appointment.

Do your research on clinics Find out what you can about the treatment options and possible clinics before contacting any of them. Find out what their success rates are for your particular situation.

Make an appointment well in advance Some clinics and consultants have long waiting lists.

Plan ahead Get blood tests and semen analysis done while you wait for your first appointment, so that you go along on the day with some information to hand. At the first consultation, have a list of questions written down. Don't be afraid of asking difficult questions and of insisting on getting clear answers if you feel unsure about what you are being told. Get a second opinion from another clinic if you are not happy with the first.

Organize your time Make sure your work fits in with any treatment, tests, and complementary therapies, not the other way round. Don't rush around between work and treatment, otherwise stress will start to affect you. Focus on finding ways to combat the inevitable stress involved when you undergo the treatment (see Steps 5 and 7 for more about stress reduction).

Eat well One of the essentials when preparing for IVF is to eat healthily. A healthy body will help with healthy eggs and sperm and will keep you strong.

Build up your reserves Sleep, relaxation techniques, and exercise are vital for building up your reserves of physical and psychological strength. Go to bed at a sensible time, get extra rest at the weekend, take up meditation or yoga, and learn a deep breathing technique (see pages 122–123). In addition, you may want to learn visualization techniques, which teach you to connect with your body, and your uterus specifically, sending positive messages of improved fertility to it. Do whatever it takes to stay relaxed on a deep level. Whatever the highs and lows of the treatment, you will be better able to cope.

Take plenty of exercise Do this in advance of starting treatment in order to help blood flow. Aerobic exercise, such as brisk 30-minute walks at least three times a week, is an excellent way of oxygenating your body and getting rid of tension (see page 88).

Manage your emotional well-being Going through the process of IVF will be emotionally draining. Be sure you have built up your reserves before you start. If you think you have any major emotional issues, seek professional help before starting treatment.

Think about who you want to tell Decide who to tell about your IVF treatment and who is mostly likely to be supportive. Negative responses from family and friends are unhelpful and can be distressing.

Q Can nutrition help with IVF?

I believe that a good diet can change the environment the eggs are in, rather than change the quality of the eggs themselves. Toxins from alcohol, cigarettes, or drugs, for example, age the ovaries, as does stress, so nutrition is very important to help counteract any harmful environmental effects. In addition, preparing nutritionally for IVF can help you to stay strong physically. It is important that you put in place all the building blocks by eating healthily before and during IVF treatment, because it can take a lot out of you. Refer back to Step 6, make sure you get plenty of omega-3 oils, and that you and your partner each take a multivitamin and mineral supplement, just to be sure.

Q Will undergoing IVF treatment affect our everyday lives?

The chances are that you and your partner lead busy, active lives, yet fertility treatment – and IVF in particular – is time consuming. This means that you need to be very practical and to plan your diary carefully. Look at the next six months and flag up any inescapable professional or social commitments you might have during that time that might interfere with treatment. Other than these, make your treatment a priority and plan your work and social commitments around it. It is very important that you do not find yourself running to appointments and scans in between meetings. In addition, you may have decided to follow certain therapies, such as acupuncture or hypnotherapy, during your treatment, and these too need to be carefully timetabled so that they leave you calmer, not more stressed. Don't take on too much, stay focused, and whatever you do in addition to your treatment, make sure it helps you to get through it, rather than cause additional pressure!

Q Is it helpful to tell other people I am doing IVF?

Emotionally, IVF is draining and feeling you are supported is key to coping with IVF. The cliché that it is an emotional roller-coaster is unfortunately true, and preparing in advance for the treatment is vital. One of the ways is to decide in advance who you are going to tell about the treatment, because there are a lot of issues attached to family and close friends, in particular. Many

women I see are worried about other people's reactions and this can create a lot of anguish. It is very common for women to tell friends, family, and colleagues, only to be met by unhelpful comments such as "What are you doing that for?" or "Stop worrying! Just relax and you'll get pregnant." Inevitably, these comments, although well-meant, are very upsetting, partly because the woman (and her partner) end up feeling misunderstood and unsupported – the very opposite of what they were hoping to get back from the person they have just told.

Think about the emotions that the people in your life create in you: go through your siblings, parents, friends, colleagues, and wider relatives, and decide who you are going to tell. Which ones can be trusted to keep the information to themselves? Which ones do you think will be unconditionally supportive and positive? Which ones are likely to come out with destructive comments? Can you anticipate suitable responses, so that they understand how you feel when they make unhelpful comments?

Don't be frightened to set boundaries with those around you. If you decide to tell them, be clear about the support you are going to need. You might have to be explicit: "I'm going to be doing this, I'm going to need your support, and I don't need you to judge me or to comment on what I'm doing." Telling someone this can actually be quite liberating because it means you are the one controlling the situation, not them.

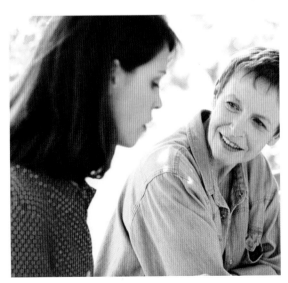

Sharing the news that you are undergoing IVF is a big step. Think carefully about who to confide in – you will need all their support.

Q Do emotions play a part in the success of IVF treatment?

In Chinese medicine (see page 133), thoughts and emotions have a huge impact on the body and, without doubt, the two main negative emotions that people suffer from when they are going through IVF are fear and guilt.

Fear, in particular, plays a large part in IVF treatment. There is the fear that women and their partners experience about telling other people, as well as the fear about how to handle other people's opinions (see page 157). There are the fears about what the treatment actually involves, about what effect the drugs will have on the woman's physical and mental health, and about what effect the treatment will have on the couple's relationship. Finally, there is the fear for many women that this is their final chance at parenthood, and that if it doesn't work they will have exhausted all the options.

Guilt – perhaps because you feel you have let down your partner or failed in some way – is the other dominant emotion for many women going through IVF. If this is a major issue and is dominating your thoughts too much, I advise you to seek professional help to help you realize that guilt should not play the part it does in your life. Men also express how guilty they feel, particularly if the reason that IVF or ICSI is needed is related to an issue with sperm. They often feel quite helpless watching their partner go through invasive treatments to counteract "their" problem.

I believe that it is possible to counteract fear and guilt: you need to see that the science of IVF is very much working for you, and that it is important to trust what the medical staff are doing, and do everything you can, including using relaxation techniques, and eating and living healthily, to contribute positively to your treatment. And the more you prepare yourself emotionally, the less energy you will waste on negative, destructive thoughts, and the more psychologically and physically resilient you will be.

Q Do you have any last-minute tips for me before I start treatment?

One week before you start IVF, I recommend couples to sit down and review the situation. Remember, you might not both be at the same stage at this point. A

case**study**

Sarah and Steve have already coped with two IVF failures. They are now taking extra measures as they prepare for their third attempt.

Sarah When the result of the pregnancy test after my second cycle of IVF was negative I was devastated. I had been so sure it was going to work. We didn't have any doubts about trying for a third time, but I knew that we had to do something different this time, even though, in theory, there seemed to be no reason why it hadn't worked.

That said, I was slightly overweight – I seemed to have gained weight after the IVF treatments – and I knew that I was incredibly stressed. The whole process is very draining and I was so desperate for it to work second time round that I think it had taken over all my thoughts. I've decided to lose some weight and have been learning relaxation techniques before I start the IVF.

Because Steve's sperm is not great we are also trying ICSI, which should improve our chances.

Steve is also making a real effort with his lifestyle and diet. We are both taking omega-3 supplements and feel we have a much more focused and planned approach.

I am going to try to take things more in my stride this time. I'm not going to overreact if I am kept waiting by the clinic and I have also decided that I am not going to talk to Steve about IVF every minute of every day – we have allocated just 10 minutes at night for this. I already feel much calmer and more in control.

Sometimes making simple changes to diet and lifestyle can be the difference between failure and success in IVF treatment.

woman might be desperate to get going, whereas her partner may be dreading the start of treatment. Spend just half an hour talking calmly about what you would like from one another. Tell each other what would help you to get through IVF, what sort of support you each need from the other. It is very important that the man voices his fears and concerns as well as the woman. Without communication that flows in both directions, fertility treatment, and IVF in particular, is a demanding, lonely road to travel down, and it can easily cause irreparable damage to a couple's relationship.

Q What if IVF doesn't work?

For the majority of couples, IVF will not work first time, as there is an element of trial and error when it comes to finding out how your body reacts to the drugs. It is better to have discussed this with your partner in advance, so that you can build in strategies for getting through the situation. The way you deal with it is to be prepared, to keep your emotional reserves as strong as possible, to communicate constantly with your partner, to communicate with – and expect answers from – the clinic that is treating you, and to control the situation as much as possible, rather than let the situation take control of you.

Allow yourselves to be upset, however, as there is no point in pretending that you are fine about the result. Many couples are devastated at each negative result, and this is perfectly normal. Don't make any hasty decisions at this stage about whether to continue or abandon future IVF treatment. Make an appointment with your clinic to analyse what may have gone wrong and to try to work out what, if anything, can/should be changed next time.

Even if you decide to stop, you should still make this appointment, if only to get some sort of closure on the entire process and to discuss whether there are any other options available to you. At my clinic, for example, we have a team who specifically offer support and advice when IVF has failed.

Q How long should I wait between treatment cycles?

When you start another treatment depends on many factors. Discuss this with your clinic, and make sure that you have allowed yourself to recover physically and mentally. I often see women who tell me they are ready

for another go at IVF, yet I can tell that mentally they are not yet ready. So listen to your head, as well as your body, before starting again, and also be advised by clinic staff.

If you are thinking of changing clinic, weigh up carefully the pros and cons of doing so, bearing in mind that you presumably chose this particular clinic originally after much thought and research.

Q What if the pregnancy test is positive?

Initially, you will no doubt be elated beyond words if a pregnancy test is positive. Soon after, though, you may be overcome by a mass of powerful and conflicting emotions. On the one hand, you will probably want to shout your news from the rooftops, on the other, you may also suddenly become anxious about what now lies ahead of you, including the almost unimaginable thought of a miscarriage. This is entirely normal and I advise all women at this stage to try to stay as calm and relaxed as possible, and to be very careful who they share their news with (see Step 10).

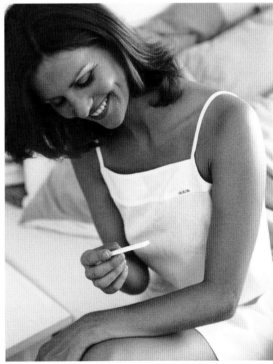

It's positive! Seeing the blue line form on a pregnancy test is a huge reward for all the efforts you have made to achieve a pregnancy.

Once you're **pregnant** there is plenty you can do to stay in **good health** for the first 12 weeks and beyond

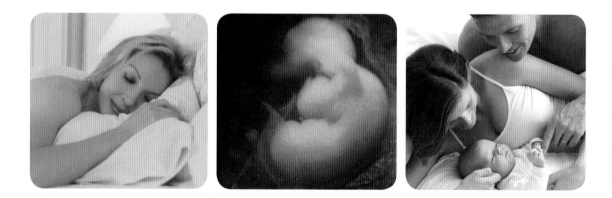

step**ten**
staying pregnant

Your questions answered on:

step 10: **staying pregnant**

It doesn't matter whether you managed to conceive naturally or using assisted conception, you will now want to do everything possible to have a **successful pregnancy** and a **healthy baby**. This chapter will help you through the **first few weeks** when many women are **at their most vulnerable**, both emotionally and physically

Q What are the key dates in pregnancy?

An average pregnancy lasts 40 weeks starting from the first day of the woman's last menstrual cycle. So if you do a pregnancy test on the day your next period is due (if yours is a 28-day cycle) and it is positive, you are four weeks pregnant.

Pregnancy is divided into three trimesters. There is a certain overlap between the time when one trimester ends and the next begins, but as a guide, the first trimester is the first 13 weeks of pregnancy; the second trimester runs from the 14th to the 28th week of pregnancy inclusive, and the third trimester runs from the 29th week to the end of the pregnancy. Because your baby is conceived about two weeks into your cycle, its gestation is two weeks behind your stage of pregnancy.

Q Is it normal to feel anxious during early pregnancy?

Many of the women I see, especially those who have been trying to conceive for a while, are at first elated when their pregnancy is confirmed and then anxious – the main worry being that they will miscarry. This is entirely normal, especially if you have conceived using IVF. Up until now you may only ever have thought of yourself as

Zita's **tip**

Learn relaxation methods in **early pregnancy** and practise them for 20 minutes every day.

someone with fertility problems who is trying to achieve a pregnancy, rather than someone who is actually carrying a baby and likely to be a parent in nine months time.

If you have had a previous miscarriage, you will probably be particularly anxious until the point at which that pregnancy ended has passed. If you are over 35, and especially if you are over 40, the chances of a first trimester miscarriage are higher, so getting to the end of the 12 weeks is also an all-important goal. All these fears are normal, particularly during the first trimester. After that time, the placenta is fully established and "takes over" the pregnancy, and the risk of miscarriage drops to only 1 per cent (see page 176).

Q We wanted this for so long. Why am I feeling doubtful now that I'm pregnant?

As well as anxiety, it is common to experience other negative emotions. You might feel panic or overwhelmed, and you may even have doubts that you really wanted this pregnancy after all. Don't feel guilty, as these emotions are the result of you becoming aware of the consequences of being pregnant. They will allow you to prepare better physically and mentally, and also to think through the practicalities of having a baby. This is your reality check and I believe these emotions are a good thing to experience.

Q Should I change my way of life now I am pregnant?

Taking good care of yourself through diet and lifestyle is the most important thing that you can do for both you and your baby. I should stress that each woman

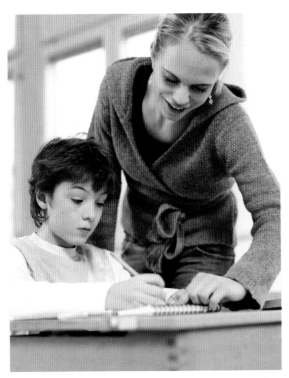

There is no need to change your life once you are pregnant: just listen to your body and slow down the pace when you need to.

is different and each pregnancy is different, so what is also important is to listen to what your body is telling you, as I believe this is nature's way of protecting your developing baby. However, it is not necessary to make drastic changes to your way of life – you can continue to work, exercise, and enjoy yourself just as you did before you became pregnant, just slow the pace a little if you are feeling tired.

Q How soon do I need to see my GP?

There is no obligation to see your GP when you first discover you are pregnant but it's a good idea to make an appointment so you can talk through any potential problems that may arise or any concerns, and discuss which screening tests and scans you want to have. You will also need to discuss the care options available to you, which vary from one Primary Care Trust to another. Generally speaking, whichever hospital you choose to give birth in – if that is where you decide to have your baby – your first appointment will be the initial "booking-in"

visit towards the end of your first trimester. This probably feels like a long way away, particularly if this is your first pregnancy. However, the sooner you see your GP, the more advance notice you will be given of the initial appointment. In the meantime, your GP can advise and support you through the initial stages of pregnancy.

Q What can I do to lay the best foundation for a healthy pregnancy?

There is no ideal way of living through pregnancy, so don't torture yourself or feel guilty if your lifestyle has sometimes fallen short of the mark. Having said that, you need to be aware that these early weeks and months are arguably the most important stages of your pregnancy so taking care of yourself (and your baby) is especially important now. What you do in the first trimester lays the building blocks for your baby's growth, because this is when all key organ and skeletal development takes place (see pages 172–175); for the growth and development of the placenta, and for your general health in pregnancy. The best way to help lay these essential foundations is to build up your reserves, both through diet and lifestyle.

Q How important is nutrition in pregnancy?

In order to grow your baby draws on your own reserves for any nutritional element that it cannot get from your daily nutrient intake. The better your diet has been before pregnancy, the better your nutritional reserves will be.

In addition, much research has been done to identify specific windows in pregnancy when you can influence key stages of your baby's development by making sure you get plenty of certain nutrients. For example, the brain and spinal cord develop from an embryonic structure called the neural tube. This starts to form by the 28th day after fertilization and it has been shown that taking a folic acid supplement before and during early pregnancy significantly reduces the incidence of neural tube defects, such as spina bifida. Another example comes in the second trimester when your baby has several growth spurts and needs a good supply of calcium. If you are not eating enough calcium-rich foods, the baby will draw on your reserves and, in so doing, will deplete your body of calcium. Similarly, if you are iron-deficient, your baby will draw on your iron reserves, leaving you anaemic and exhausted.

Q How can I make a **healthy start**?

During the first trimester, not only will the foundations be laid for the development of all your baby's organs, but also for you to stay strong and be able to nurture a growing baby. There are plenty of things you can do to help both of you stay healthy through the first 12 weeks of pregnancy and beyond.

Rest Getting plenty of rest is always top of my list of recommended things to do. Pregnancy, especially in the first trimester, can leave you absolutely exhausted, particularly towards the end of the day (see page 171). Listen to your body: if it is telling you it needs to sleep when you get back from work, don't ignore it. Go to bed, even for a couple of hours until dinner. And make sure you don't have to cook the meal yourself!

Give up cigarettes today The toxins from cigarettes cross the placenta and harm the developing fetus at all stages of pregnancy. Smoking is a known factor in miscarriage because it deprives the placenta of oxygen. It also reduces oxygen supply to the fetus.

Stop drinking alcohol Alcohol is toxic to the fetus. It also reduces the oxygen flow to the placenta, thus affecting fetal development. I advise that women drink no alcohol at all during pregnancy.

Avoid coffee High caffeine consumption is known to raise the risk of miscarriage (see pages 176–177). Fortunately, nature usually takes care of the problem because many women go off coffee entirely during the first three months of pregnancy.

Avoid doing strenuous exercise This includes exercise involving bouncing such as horseriding or trampolining. Exercise in itself is good during pregnancy (see pages 168–169) but, once again, I believe you should listen to what your body is telling you. Often, during the first three months, women feel too sick and exhausted to do anything other than gentle exercise. If you have conceived with IVF, I don't recommend doing any exercise during the first trimester.

Avoid hot baths and saunas or steam rooms These should be avoided as they can raise the body temperature and this could be damaging to the developing embryo or fetus.

Learn to relax If you haven't done so already, you need to slow down your pace of life and avoid rushing around for the first trimester. Minimize stress in your life by making use of relaxation exercises and techniques (see pages 122–123).

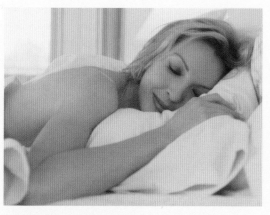

Getting plenty of rest is essential when it comes to coping with pregnancy, especially in the first trimester.

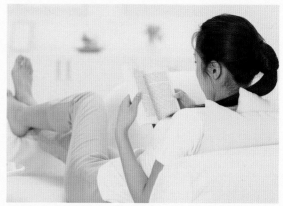

Relaxation is key. Take time out of your busy routine to simply sit still and read a book or, even better, do nothing.

Adopt a healthy eating plan It takes time in the early stages of pregnancy to establish your healthy eating plan, bearing in mind you may be feeling nauseous or you may have cravings for certain foods. Try to follow the advice on page 167, as good nutrition is key in the first trimester.

Stop taking any pre-pregnancy supplements Switch to a specific pregnancy multivitamin and mineral supplement and make sure you are taking a minimum of 400mcg of folic acid. Even if you weren't taking this before getting pregnant, it's not too late to start now. If you only take one supplement, take this one. Under certain circumstances, some women may be prescribed a higher dose.

Avoid sex If you have a history of miscarriage, of first trimester bleeding, or if you have conceived using IVF you should avoid having sex during the first trimester. You will need to explain this to your partner and to try and find ways of staying physically intimate during this time. Again, because of the symptoms of early pregnancy, such as nausea and exhaustion (see pages 170–171), many women lose their libido anyway during these early weeks. If this has happened to you, do take time to communicate the reasons to your partner.

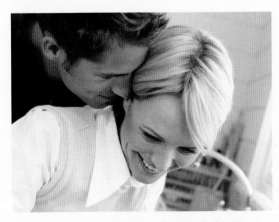

You may have been advised to avoid sex in the first trimester, but you can still enjoy a loving relationship with your partner.

Q Is it a good idea to take a multivitamin and mineral supplement?

What you eat – and more especially what you have eaten in the three to four months before getting pregnant – will impact on your well-being and that of your baby. However, during the first trimester in particular, I believe that it is also a good idea to take a multivitamin and mineral supplement aimed specifically at pregnancy to counteract any deficiencies you may have during the first 12 weeks. This is the time when women's eating patterns are often haywire due to nausea or vomiting. The supplement will also make sure you receive enough of the antioxidant vitamins and minerals, including vitamins C and E, selenium, and co-enzyme Q10, all of which are important for placental health and cell growth in the embryo. A fish oil supplement contains omega-3 and omega-6 essential fatty acids, which are important for development of your baby's brain, eyes, and nerve cells.

Q What are the key rules for eating well in early pregnancy?

Your energy needs will vary from day to day and from one part of your pregnancy to another. Your calorie intake in the first trimester should be no different from your intake before you were pregnant ("eating for two" is a myth), and indeed if you are within the normal BMI range (see page 13), your weight gain should only be around 2kg (4lb 6oz) during this time. However, you will slowly start to recognize how much to eat and when, as your body starts to tell you what its needs are.

This is complicated by the fact that, in the first trimester, many women suffer from nausea and vomiting and a few suffer from this throughout their pregnancy. Doctors still do not know why some women are affected by these symptoms but one theory is that low blood sugar levels may be at least partly responsible. For some women the symptoms are worse in the morning (after many hours without food) and for others they are worse in the evening when they are tired and their blood sugar levels may have also started to dip.

Whether or not you are affected by nausea or vomiting (see page 171 for how to cope) there are certain rules that you should try to stick to when it comes to establishing a healthy diet throughout pregnancy (see page 167).

Q I'm a vegetarian. Do I need a special diet during pregnancy?

If you are vegetarian, you need to pay particular attention to your intake of protein, vitamin B_{12}, calcium, and iron. You can do this by making sure you eat plenty of:

- nuts
- pulses (such as chickpeas, peas, and beans)
- dairy foods (such as cottage cheese and semi-skimmed milk – fruit smoothies are a great source of nutrients)
- eggs.

Zinc is especially important in pregnancy as it plays a role in cell division and helps to form your baby's immune system. Good sources include wholegrains, cereals, and seeds.

If you are vegan, you should speak to your doctor as you may need to take supplements to ensure you get the right intake of these nutrients.

Smoothies rich in fruit can combine the benefits of low-fat milk with the vitamins, minerals, and fibre provided by the fruit.

Q Which foods should I avoid?

Women are now bombarded with so much advice concerning what they should and shouldn't eat in pregnancy that it is easy to become unduly anxious. The following foods may pose a risk to your well-being and that of your baby and you are advised to avoid them in pregnancy. However, I want to stress that if you have eaten any of the foods below you should not panic.

- Unpasteurized or blue cheeses (including brie, camembert, gorgonzola) and pâtés may contain listeria, a rare bacterium that can have potentially fatal consequences for your unborn baby.
- Cooked meats and pâtés can also contain *E.coli*, another rare but potentially dangerous bacterium.
- Raw fish and shellfish, raw or undercooked eggs, and raw or undercooked meat (especially chicken) can contain salmonella, a bacterium that is killed by heat. Salmonella infection causes unpleasant symptoms in the mother but it does not cross the placenta, so the baby is not affected.
- Chilled foods and ready-washed bagged salads. These can contain listeria or salmonella.
- Raw or undercooked meat and unwashed fruit and vegetables may be infected with toxoplasmosis, a parasitic infection carried in cat faeces, which can cause damage to the fetus. Eighty per cent of the population is already infected (and immune), and toxoplasmosis is only potentially dangerous if infection occurs for the first time during the first trimester. Always wash fruit and vegetables thoroughly and wash your hands after handling these and raw meat.
- Liver contains high levels of vitamin A, which has been linked to fetal abnormality.
- Large predatory fish, such as tuna or swordfish, can contain high levels of mercury, and farmed salmon may contain high levels of pesticides.

Q I am craving carbs but worry I will put on too much weight. What should I do?

Women often worry when they start to crave a lot of carbohydrate in the first trimester but this is perfectly normal, as you need energy. The key is to eat little and often and to make sure you eat plenty of "good carbs" (see page 102) rather than snacking on lots of sugary, refined, or processed foods. Use organic honey or jams made without extra sugar and eat organic chocolate when you need a sweet "fix".

Q What key things should I keep in mind when planning a **pregnancy eating plan**?

Don't become obsessive over what you eat while you are pregnant. Instead, just try to employ the following simple rules.

Eat little and often This will keep your blood sugar levels balanced. As your pregnancy progresses, your stomach will find it easier if presented with small meals to digest.

Mix protein and carbohydrate This helps to keep your blood sugar levels balanced.

Cut down on fatty foods This is especially important if you suffer from nausea and vomiting.

Avoid hydrogenated fats These are found in margarine and processed food and avoid saturated fats (found in butter and fatty cuts of meat).

Eat lean protein This is easily digestible: chicken, fish, and pulses are good sources, as is semi-skimmed milk and cottage cheese.

Eat oily fish Oily fish, such as wild salmon and trout, are rich in omega-3 EFAs, which are important for fetal brain development. Eat them twice a week.

Avoid simple carbs (see page 102) If you crave something sweet, eat organic 85 per cent cocoa chocolate and snacks containing slow-releasing carbs, such as oat biscuits, dried apricots, and figs.

Eat a wide variety of (ideally, seasonal) fruit and vegetables These will provide you with many different vitamins and minerals, which will give you essential nutrients and sufficient fibre (the bowel often becomes sluggish during pregnancy). Fruit and vegetables are also a great source of antioxidants, which are important in pregnancy as they protect the fetus from exposure to free radicals in the mother's bloodstream. Follow the government recommendation and eat five portions a day.

Steam, bake, sweat or stir-fry foods This will preserve their nutritional value as much as possible.

Reduce your salt intake to a minimum to avoid fluid retention.

Avoid food additives whenever possible.

Drink at least 1.5 litres (2½ pints) of filtered water a day Herbal teas are also good.

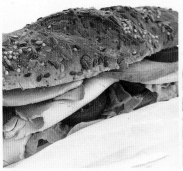

A chicken salad sandwich provides a good range of nutrients.

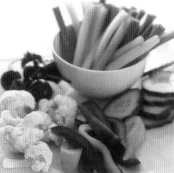

A rainbow diet ensures you are getting all the vitamins and minerals you need.

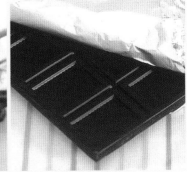

Organic chocolate with a high cocoa percentage can help beat sweet cravings.

Q Is it safe to exercise during early pregnancy?

This is a difficult question to answer because the same answer doesn't apply to all women. Ultimately, I believe that your body will tell you how much exercise you can and should be doing and that, often, the early pregnancy symptoms of nausea, vomiting, and tiredness are enough to stop many women doing too much. Even those women who are used to exercising regularly may find that for the first three months they do nothing other than a bit of gentle walking, and that is absolutely fine. I don't believe in forcing yourself to move around when you are physically exhausted or feeling sick. Indeed, I think this is part of nature's way of telling you to take it easy. You will feel much more energized as you reach the end of the first trimester, and will find you can start to exercise once again.

However, if you feel up to exercising during the first three months and you did so regularly before getting pregnant, I would advise you to continue doing what you feel comfortable with, albeit at a slower, less intense level. I would, however, recommend that you give up running, trampolining, or horse riding, as these involve repetitive bouncing. If you regularly go to an aerobics class, tell the instructor you are pregnant and be sure to take it easy. If you go to the gym, avoid doing abdominal exercises and use lighter weights, as you could damage tendons and ligaments during pregnancy (they become looser in preparation for birth, so you should avoid putting too much pressure on them). Make use of aerobic machines such as rowing machines, treadmills, and bikes, as these do not involve bouncing.

Whatever exercise you choose, be aware of the following:
- Don't get too hot or out of breath.
- Don't let your heart rate go over 140 beats per minute.

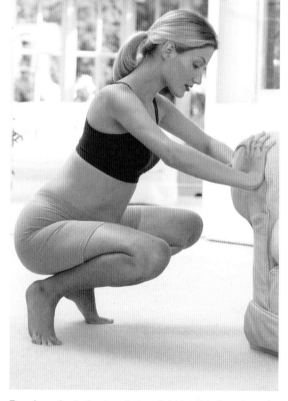

Exercise only at a level you feel comfortable with in the early weeks of pregnancy. Don't worry if you don't feel like exercising at all.

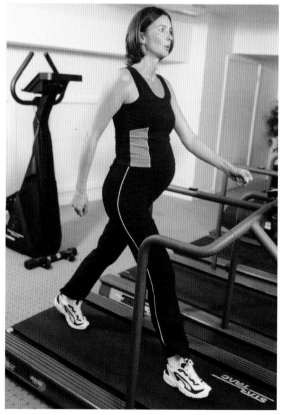

If you were used to exercising before you became pregnant, keep it up, but at a less intense level.

- Don't do strenuous exercise for more than 15 minutes at a time.
- Cool down for the same amount of time at the end.
- If you experience any pain, dizziness, or faintness stop at once.

If you don't exercise regularly, now is not the time to start doing anything other than gentle exercise, such as walking, yoga, or specific pregnancy exercise classes under the supervision of a teacher who understands the physiological changes in pregnancy.

If you are a high-risk pregnancy (for example, you used assisted conception, especially IVF, or have had a previous miscarriage, or are over 35), I would advise you not to exercise at all during the first trimester, just in case.

Q What are the benefits of exercise in early pregnancy?

Exercise is good for you throughout pregnancy, as long as you do not overdo things. It will give you more energy and will keep you strong and supple, which will help you through pregnancy and during labour and birth.

If you are a regular exerciser, you will already be more toned and have greater endurance, and this too will help you later on. Your blood volume increases if you exercise and you boost circulation and oxygen levels, and this helps to promote fetal growth.

In addition, exercise helps make you feel more positive and prevents depression as natural mood-enhancing chemicals called endorphins are released in the brain.

Q Since I discovered I was pregnant, I've been feeling very anxious and stressed at work. What can I do to make things better?

You are probably feeling a little overwhelmed by everything and this is not uncommon, particularly as you make adjustments to your life in the early stages of pregnancy. Build time into each day for relaxation and breathing exercises and make going to bed early a priority. This will help you to regain a sense of control. If you feel up to it, light exercise can also help to relieve stress and tension – try to make sure you leave the office at lunchtime and go for a walk.

case**study**

Carol has just reached the end of the first trimester of her first pregnancy. She became pregnant after trying to conceive for 14 months.

Carol I wasn't expecting to feel anxious when my pregnancy test proved positive – I had always assumed I would just be ecstatically happy when that happened. But after the initial excitement wore off I found I began to worry and I became very aware of every twinge, ache, and pain I felt. I then started to have some spotting, which totally panicked me.

My job is very busy and involves a lot of driving, but I didn't want to have to tell my boss I was pregnant because it was still very early days. I was so relieved when I could go and see Anita O'Neill at the Zita West Clinic for an early pregnancy consultation. She helped me to work out a plan of action and that helped me to feel more in control. She also arranged an early scan and this reassured me that all was well. I started to relax a little.

After the scan, I had a chat with my boss and we agreed I should cut back on the amount of driving I was doing. I have also been learning some breathing techniques, which help me to cope when I feel worried. At last, I feel I am really beginning to connect with my baby.

I have now passed the all-important 12-week milestone and have started to tell my family, friends, and more of my colleagues. It's been a long journey and I still have some way to go but I'm beginning to believe that I am going to be a mum.

When pregnancy finally happens it can be very scary. Seek reassurance and do all you can to make sure you stay relaxed and enjoy each stage.

Q What are the normal side effects of early pregnancy?

One of the most worrying things in the first trimester, particularly if you have never been pregnant before, is deciding whether each twinge or episode of dizziness is something to be concerned about.

The fact is that most women will experience a variety of symptoms, ranging from swollen, aching breasts to tiredness and nausea, during the first 12 weeks (see below), while their bodies adapt to being pregnant. As ever, each woman will have a different experience from other women and also from one pregnancy to the next. Generally, though, even those who are not overwhelmed by early pregnancy symptoms, say that they nonetheless "feel" pregnant in an indefinable way.

In the vast majority of cases, side effects are to be expected and are nothing to worry about. However, if you have any persistent bleeding or intense abdominal pain or cramps, then you should either go to see your GP or go to your hospital to find out whether there is anything wrong.

Q Can nausea or vomiting cause problems in pregnancy?

Only a very few women are so debilitated by nausea and vomiting over a period of weeks, rather than days, that they cannot keep down fluids or food and so become weak and dehydrated. These women may need to be admitted to hospital until their fluid, glucose, and mineral levels have been restored. However, for most women, being unable to eat or drink properly is

Q What are common **pregnancy concerns**?

Many women sail through their pregnancy with few concerns or complications. However, it is not uncommon to experience some symptoms, especially in the early stages.

Tiredness It is not unusual to feel tired. Listen to your body and rest as much as you can.

Breast tenderness This affects some women more than others. It is caused by hormones, including high levels of oestrogen.

Nausea and vomiting These are common, but absence of these symptoms is by no means a sign that your pregnancy is not progressing normally.

A need to urinate more frequently This is caused by increased blood supply and therefore increased volume being filtered by the kidneys.

Dizziness and feeling faint Can be caused by low blood sugar levels, especially if you are not eating properly, or by blood pooling in your legs and not reaching your brain sufficiently. If symptoms keep occurring, consult your doctor.

Abdominal pain Some aches and pains in the lower abdomen are common and are usually a sign that your pelvic ligaments and muscles are being forced to move and stretch as a result of your gradually expanding uterus. However, if the ache feels more like a constant pain, or increases in severity, go to see your doctor immediately, especially if you are in the first eight weeks of pregnancy. It is possible that you have an ectopic pregnancy (see page 26) and if this is the case, you will need urgent treatment.

Bleeding This is the single most feared early pregnancy symptom, as it can indicate the start of a miscarriage. However, as many as one in three women have some sort of bleeding in the first trimester, and most go on to carry their pregnancy to term.

Bleeding can range from a little brown bleeding to light red spotting to passing large blood clots, yet any of these can be harmless. However, you should investigate any episode of bleeding, particularly if it is bright red or if you have passed clots. Your local hospital can usually arrange for an ultrasound scan and, as early as the sixth week of pregnancy, a doctor will be able to identify a problem or reassure you that your pregnancy is developing normally.

Zita's **tip**

Build **relaxation** into your routine and build up your **reserves of sleep** throughout pregnancy.

Q Is it normal to feel so exhausted?

As with morning sickness, no one really understands why it is that so many women feel so tired during the early weeks of pregnancy. Some doctors believe that the rapid changes taking place in your body and your metabolism in response to your pregnancy are simply tiring you out. Another explanation is that it is due to the speed of development of the embryo inside you. (Again, I must stress that if you don't feel overly tired you should not worry – every pregnancy is different and it is even common for the same woman to feel exhausted in one pregnancy and absolutely fine in another.)

This lack of energy can be very debilitating and rather overwhelming for many women, but it is important to understand that it is perfectly normal and whatever the reason for these feelings, rest and sleep are essential. Take catnaps during the day, or longer siestas if you can, and go to bed earlier at night.

In general, any feelings of lethargy or tiredness disappear by the end of the first trimester, after which women often find they are once again full of energy.

no more than an unpleasant, temporary side effect of pregnancy and it poses no danger to the health of their developing baby. Whatever your daily intake, your baby will be taking its nutrients from your existing reserves (see page 163).

Let me reassure you that, in the vast majority of cases, symptoms of nausea and sickness pass by the end of the first trimester, and as soon as you feel better, you will start to replenish those reserves so that you and your baby will have the nutrition you both need in the weeks and months ahead.

I should also emphasize that *not* feeling sick is not a sign that something is wrong either. Some fortunate women are entirely unaffected by sickness and this has no bearing whatsoever on their overall pregnancy.

Q What are the best ways to cope with morning sickness?

There is no magic remedy to get rid of the unpleasant symptoms of morning sickness – which can, in fact, strike at any time of day. However, some of the following tips may help you to cope:

- Eat little and often.
- Avoid fatty or spicy foods.
- Eat bland easy-to-digest food. Foods such as dry biscuits, rice cakes, and porridge (mixed if possible with skimmed or semi-skimmed milk) are good.
- Peppermint tea combats the metallic taste in the mouth caused by nausea.
- Ginger (for example, in the form of ginger tea, ginger capsules, crystallized ginger, or ginger biscuits) is often helpful in alleviating symptoms of nausea.
- If sickness is worse in the morning, try eating a dry biscuit first thing, before you get out of bed.
- Acupuncture has been shown to help in relieving the symptoms of morning sickness. Some women use an acupressure wristband that presses on the acupuncture point on the inside of the wrist.

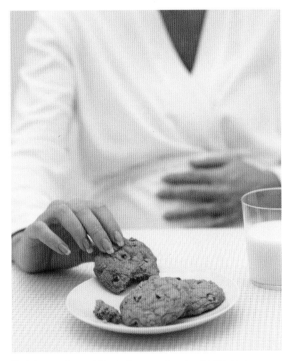

If sickness does strike in the morning, try nibbling on a biscuit to boost blood sugar levels before you face the day.

find out more: **the first 13 weeks**

The first trimester is the most important in terms of laying the foundation for a healthy pregnancy, both for you and your developing baby.

By the end of the 13th week, the tiny cluster of cells that embedded in your uterus at the start of pregnancy is already a fully formed human being. All the major organs are in place and your pregnancy is no longer supported by complex hormonal interactions, but by the fully established placenta instead.

your baby and body at 0–6 weeks

Your baby By the time the fertilized egg has started to divide, travelled down the fallopian tube, and embedded in the endometrium, or uterine lining, the resulting cluster of cells numbers around 60 and is called a blastocyst. This process has taken around three days.

▨ After another two to three days, the blastocyst has fully embedded in the endometrium and has subdivided further to around 100 cells. There are two distinct layers of cells by now: the outer layer, called trophoblast cells, which will become the placenta; and the inner cells, which will develop into the embryo.

▨ This inner mass of cells further specializes during the second week after conception into three types of cells. Each type develops into a different part of the body: the outer layer, or ectoderm, forms the skin, hair, nails, tooth enamel, and also, crucially, the brain and nervous system. The middle layer, or mesoderm, forms the skeleton, muscles, kidneys, heart, blood vessels, and reproductive organs. The inner layer, or endoderm, forms the respiratory and digestive systems, as well as the bladder and urinary tract. So it is that, even before you even know you are pregnant, a huge amount of development has taken place and the key parts of your baby's body are starting to form.

▨ By the end of week 6, the embryo measures around 4mm in length, weighs less than 1g (0.03oz), and resembles a tadpole or a comma. It has folded in on itself, and a bulge in the middle represents the beginnings of a heart, which starts to "flutter" and pulse, like a heart beat.

▨ A structure called the neural tube starts to form into what will become the spinal cord at the lower end, enveloped by a rudimentary spinal column, and the brain at the upper end. Nerve cells form the various folds and hollows that will develop into the different parts of the brain. The beginnings of a mouth and eyes are almost visible.

▨ The embryo floats in a bubble-like fluid-filled sac, the amniotic sac, which protects it from the outside world. It receives its sustenance from a balloon-like structure called a yolk-sac, attached to it by a stalk. The outer part of the amniotic sac is called the chorion and part of this will eventually become the placenta.

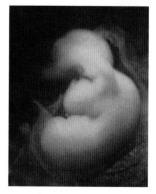

After 28 days development, the most primitive embryonic organ systems are formed.

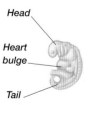

Head

Heart bulge

Tail

By six weeks gestation all the heart cells are beating as one and the basic fetal nervous system is in place.

Your body When the blastocyst embeds in the uterine lining, it starts to secrete human chorionic gonadotrophin (hCG), which in turn tells the corpus luteum (the tissue mass formed by the follicle after the egg has been released from it) to secrete progesterone to help keep the embryo in place. This hormone also thickens your cervical mucus to form a plug, which seals off your uterus. Raised levels of oestrogen have also helped to thicken the endometrium to allow the embryo to embed. If the level of either of these hormones drops in the first trimester, the pregnancy will end in miscarriage.

By the end of the sixth week your uterus, which was about the size of a plum, has expanded to the size of an apple.

Your metabolic rate will increase by as much as 10 to 25 per cent to allow the production of suffcient oxygen to reach all the tissues of all your organs. By the end of the sixth week, the blood supply to your uterus has doubled. Your uterus has started to expand and your blood volume has started to increase to ensure that it can fill all the newly formed blood vessels in the uterus and, eventually, the placenta. All your major organs will receive a boost in blood flow during pregnancy. Because the volume of blood increases from about 5 litres (8¾ pints) to around 7 to 8 litres (12 to 14 pints), the number of red blood cells also needs to rise. This is why maintaining a good intake of iron-rich foods is so important.

your baby and body at 6–10 weeks

Your baby From around the eighth week the embryo is referred to as a fetus. By the end of the 10th week, it measures 30mm (1¼in) and weighs 3 to 5g (0.1oz).
■ The neck and forehead start to develop, and the eyes start to move to the front of the head. Toothbuds that will form the milk teeth are in place in the jawbone.
■ The limb buds are now developing into limbs and webbed hands become separate fingers by the end of week 10.
■ The little tail has almost completely disappeared.
■ Vertebrae develop on each side of the spinal column and the increasingly complex nervous system evolves. The fetus can be seen making small, jerky movements.
■ By 10 weeks, the heart's four chambers are visible on an ultrasound scan. It pumps blood through the fast-developing circulatory system at around 180 beats per minute, twice the normal adult resting heartrate.
■ The stomach, liver, kidneys, and other parts of the digestive system are all in place.

■ The amniotic sac's outer layer, or chorion, begins to develop finger-like projections called villi, and these become concentrated on one side, burrowing into the uterine wall with the help of newly formed blood vessels. These villi will eventually form the placenta, which will protect your baby. However, the fetus is still vulnerable to toxins (see page 176).

Your body Your metabolic rate has increased. Pregnancy hormones relax your muscles, including your heart muscle. The blood vessels also relax (become more dilated) to allow a greater volume of blood to be pumped around your body without your blood pressure rising to dangerous levels.

The skin around your nipples (the areola) will probably be darker than usual thanks to the increase in blood flow and blood volume. Your breasts have started to swell and are much more tender because the milk ducts are beginning to prepare themselves for lactation at the end of pregnancy.

Brain
Eye
Arm
Umbilical cord
Leg

Between six and eight weeks, the fetus is developing facial features that are recognizably human.

At eight weeks the fetus is approximately 25mm (1in) in length.

your baby and body at 10–13 weeks

Your baby By the end of the 13th week, all the major fetal organs, muscles, and bones have been formed.

■ Elbows, wrists, and hands are clearly visible, and the lower limbs are also continuing to develop.

■ Calcium deposits in the limbs and teeth begin the process of bone formation (ossification) by the 12th week. This continues until birth, although the actual hardening of the skeleton will not cease until adolescence.

■ The fetus will have a reflex response to an outside stimulus, so if the mother's abdomen is prodded, it will try to move away.

■ The fetus' ovaries or testes are fully formed, although external genitalia (the penis and clitoris) are not yet distinguishable.

■ The fetal blood is gradually being manufactured by its liver, rather than the yolk sac.

Placenta

Amniotic fluid

Fingers and toes *are no longer webbed*

At 13 weeks the rapidly developing nervous system and limbs allow the fetus to move freely.

Your body By the end of the first trimester, about one quarter of your cardiac output (the amount of blood pumped around your body) will be directed towards your uterus, compared to only 2 per cent in your non-pregnant state. You may find that you occasionally feel breathless as your lungs adapt to take in an increased amount of oxygen with every breath.

If you have been suffering from tiredness and sickness these symptoms should start to diminish now. You will be able to start eating normally again and will soon be back to feeling like your old self.

Your waist will probably have thickened slightly and you will have put on a little weight. Your breasts will continue to develop. As your uterus enlarges and the ligaments attaching it to the side of your pelvis are stretched, you may experience an occasional ache or twinge.

By the 13th week your baby is 80mm (3in) long and weighs 25g (about 1oz).

the placenta

By the end of the 13th week, your pregnancy is no longer supported by your hormones but by the fully established placenta instead. The placenta acts as the lungs and kidneys of the fetus. Between the placenta and the fetus runs the umbilical cord, which consists of a large vein carrying oxygenated blood and nutrients from the mother to the baby and two small arteries carrying waste products and de-oxygenated blood back to the mother from the fetus. The fetal and maternal circulations are separated by a thin membrane and never mix, which is why the placenta acts as a barrier, preventing the passage of most harmful substances from

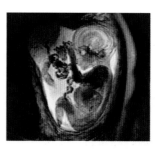

Mature placenta The placenta grows rapidly to supply all the baby's needs throughout pregnancy. By the end of the third trimester, it measures 20–25cm (8–10in) in diameter and weighs around 700g (1½lb).

the mother to the fetus (see page 176). Even if there is blood loss from the mother, or the placenta is damaged, the fetal circulation is protected.

your 12-week scan

Between 11 and 13 weeks you will be offered a routine ultrasound scan, which helps to monitor fetal growth and development. This will also be used to confirm your baby's estimated date of delivery (EDD).

Ultrasound scans work by sending high-frequency sound waves through your body using a small, handheld probe called a transducer. Echoes produced as the pulses strike structures are converted into electrical signals, which are processed to produce an image. Before you have an abdominal ultrasound scan you will be asked to drink several pints of water and to avoid emptying your bladder. Your expanded bladder reduces the space in the lower abdomen and pushes the uterus upwards, making it easier for the sonographer to get a clear image. He or she will take key measurements – the circumference of the head and abdomen and length of the femur (thigh bone) – and the relationship between these gives an indication of growth. Your baby's heartbeat will also be monitored and you will be able to see it beating fast on the screen.

Ultrasound scans can detect most fetal abnormalities and they identify disorders that might put the baby at risk. Not everything can be picked up by a scan, but the detection rate for anencephaly (brain defect), for example, is 98 per cent, and for spina bifida it is 80 per cent. Screening is done for all types of chromosomal disorders, in particular Down's syndrome (see below).

Multiple pregnancies are often diagnosed during the 12-week scan, although they can be detected earlier if you have a six-week scan (usually following IVF treatment) when two or more fetal sacs will be visible in the uterus.

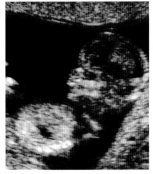

This 3D ultrasound scan is of a 12-week-old fetus in the uterus. Its head is on the right, and the developing facial features can be seen.

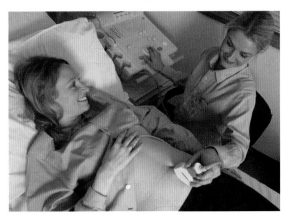

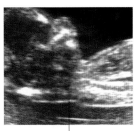

The sonographer sweeps a hand-held transducer across your abdomen to pick up sound waves from fetal structures.

nuchal translucency scan

During your 12-week scan, measurements will also be taken to establish the amount of fluid under the skin at the back of the baby's neck – the nuchal translucency. This is used to establish whether there is an increased risk of the baby having Down's syndrome. Less than 3mm of fluid behind the neck indicates a low risk, and this will be the result for 95 per cent of women. If the measurement is between 4 and 7mm, further investigations will be offered. The nuchal scan gives an indication of the possibility of Down's syndrome but is by no means conclusive and relies on further diagnostic tests, such as amniocentesis, to confirm the diagnosis.

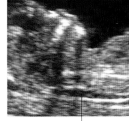

Normal fluid

The small depth of fluid behind the neck indicates a low risk of Down's syndrome.

Increased fluid

A larger depth of fluid puts the fetus at a higher risk of Down's syndrome.

Q Which medicines can I take safely in pregnancy?

Many medicines – even over-the-counter remedies – are not recommended during pregnancy, although fortunately if you have taken any without knowing you were pregnant, they are unlikely to have had any harmful effect on the fetus. However, you should always check with your doctor if a particular prescription drug can be taken during pregnancy, and check with a pharmacist if you are buying a non-prescription drug. Even if they are technically safe, you may find that some medications (such as indigestion remedies) affect absorption of vitamins and minerals, so it is best not to take them unless strictly necessary.

Q Are **infections** a risk in pregnancy?

Many women worry that an infection might affect their pregnancy, but I can reassure you that infections such as the common cold, 'flu, throat infections, gastroenteritis, and general tummy upsets are not dangerous for your pregnancy or your baby. However, if you have been exposed to diseases such as chickenpox, rubella (see page 14), or measles and you have not had the disease yourself or have not been immunized this can be a cause for concern and you should consult your GP.

Chickenpox This is a highly contagious virus that is extremely common among young children, but which is unlikely to affect your pregnancy or your baby if you catch it. If you contract chickenpox during the first 8 weeks of pregnancy, it is unlikely to cause you to miscarry or to affect the embryo. If you contract it between weeks 8 and 20, there is only a very small risk (1–2 per cent) of it affecting your baby.

Measles One of the most contagious viral diseases, and if contracted during pregnancy measles can lead to miscarriage and to infection of your unborn baby. In the worst cases, it can result in the death of the baby if infection occurs near delivery date.

Q Are herbal medicines safe to take in pregnancy?

Some herbal remedies can interfere with fetal development, just as traditional medication can. You must consult a qualified herbalist before taking any herbal remedy whatsoever during pregnancy but be aware that herbal medicines are not subject to rigorous clinical trials in the way that conventional medicines are. Just because a remedy is "natural", it doesn't mean it is harmless or automatically good for you!

Q What else might harm my baby?

Harmful substances that can cross the placental barrier and therefore affect the embryo or fetus are called teratogens. Exposure to teratogens during the first trimester, when vital organ development (organogenesis) is taking place, can lead to birth defects. Common and known teratogens include:
- certain medications, such as sedatives, antidepressants, anti-malarial drugs, and some herbal remedies
- recreational drugs, such as marijuana and cocaine,
- nicotine and alcohol
- chemicals, such as lead, PCBs, and dioxins
- radiation, as in X-rays.

Q What are the chances of me having a miscarriage in the first 12 weeks?

Miscarriage is the most common pregnancy problem, but the vast majority occur very early on, often before you even know you are pregnant.
- At six weeks, approximately 1 in 6 pregnancies, or 15 per cent, will end in miscarriage.
- At eight weeks, the odds of the pregnancy ending in a miscarriage have fallen dramatically to around 1 in 16 pregnancies, or 6 per cent.
- After 12 weeks of pregnancy, only 1 per cent of pregnancies end in miscarriage.

Q Why does miscarriage happen?

The vast majority of miscarriages are due to a chromosomal abnormality that makes it impossible for the fetus to survive. The risks of chromosomal anomalies do increase with age, but otherwise, these so-called random miscarriages are simply down to "bad luck". Occasionally, there is a hormonal or physical reason why a woman miscarries (such as a uterine abnormality or a weak cervix). Smoking increases the risk of miscarriage and having a previous miscarriage raises the chances of having another one. In a very small number of women, there is an autoimmune problem, which causes recurrent miscarriages. Infections such as listeria, rubella, and some STIs can also cause a pregnancy to end.

However, despite what you may have been told, the following do not cause miscarriages: normal exercising, lack of rest, lifting, eating spicy food, sex, travel, sitting at a computer screen, and constipation. In some instances, they may not be good for pregnancy, but babies are well protected in the uterine environment, and, unless you are a high-risk pregnancy, you should carry on as normal and aim to have as healthy a diet and lifestyle as possible.

Q How will I cope if I do have a miscarriage?

If you are unlucky enough to miscarry, you must not blame yourself, as it is unlikely that anything you did contributed to the pregnancy loss. Losing a baby at any stage of pregnancy is devastating and it can take several months to recover physically and, especially, mentally. Your acute sense of loss means that mourning and grief will go through various stages, from shock and disbelief, to numbness, confusion, anger, guilt, and maybe even depression. Don't hesitate to seek specialist professional help for both psychological and medical care: many maternity units will have counsellors who are trained to help you and your partner come to terms with what you have gone through.

Whether or not you tell family, friends, and colleagues (who may not even have known you were pregnant) will be a personal decision, but one which you might be helped to reach with professional guidance. You will also be helped to decide how long to wait before trying for another baby. Make sure that when you do start again you are strong enough both physically and mentally.

Q We have reached the end of the first trimester. Are we really going to be parents?

Getting through the first 12 weeks of pregnancy is always seen as a major step for women, especially those who have had problems getting or staying pregnant. After

this time, the pregnancy is no longer supported by hormones, but by the placenta, and the risk of miscarriage falls dramatically. Women who miscarry after the first trimester do so either because their baby has a congenital abnormality (which is often genetic in origin), or because they have contracted an infection such as listeria, or because their body is physically not able to carry a pregnancy. Luckily, such cases are rare, so once the 12th week has passed, couples usually feel sufficiently relaxed and confident about the pregnancy to be able to tell family and friends about it.

There are sound reasons for believing that you can now start to enjoy the rest your pregnancy, safe in the knowledge that it is unlikely that anything will go wrong. You can begin to plan in more concrete terms for the arrival of your baby in a few months' time.

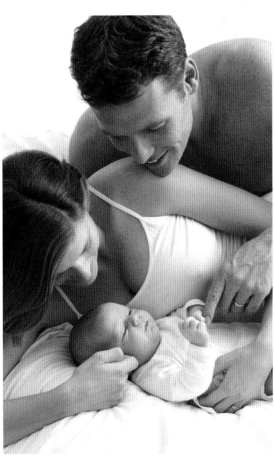

Your future as parents becomes more assured now that the generally more hazardous first trimester has passed.

questionnaire: **early pregnancy**

Great news! **You are pregnant** and may already be experiencing some of the highs and lows of the first few weeks of pregnancy. This questionnaire is a little different: you score 1 for every "yes" to check you are doing all you can **to manage the early stages** and to ensure **the healthiest possible start** for your baby

1 Are you using relaxation techniques to reduce any stress and anxieties you might have?
yes ☐ **no** ☐
It is normal to feel worried and to have mixed emotions when you discover you are pregnant. Try to stay as relaxed as possible and to keep your reserves of energy as full as possible.

2 Are you going to bed earlier than normal?
yes ☐ **no** ☐
Many women feel tired during the first trimester, and it is important to make sure you get extra sleep in order to cope with the extra demands that early pregnancy is making on your body.

3 Are you resting if you feel like it during the day?
yes ☐ **no** ☐
It can be difficult to accept that you may have to rest during the day, but listen to what your body is telling you. Your energy reserves are important.

4 Are you taking a daily folic acid supplement (400mcg)?
yes ☐ **no** ☐
If you take only one vitamin supplement, make sure it is this one.

5 Are you taking a specific pregnancy multivitamin and mineral supplement?
yes ☐ **no** ☐
A supplement can be useful in the first trimester when morning sickness can make it difficult to eat well (see page 165).

6 Are you exercising?
yes ☐ **no** ☐
If you are not a high-risk pregnancy, exercise is good for you in early pregnancy (see pages 168–169).

7 Have you given up smoking and drinking alcohol?
yes ☐ **no** ☐
Both of these affect the baby, as their toxic elements cross the placenta and reduce the oxygen the baby receives.

8 Have you given up caffeine?
yes ☐ **no** ☐
High caffeine consumption has been linked to an increased risk of miscarriage.

9 Have you cut the potentially harmful foods listed on page 166 out of your diet?
yes ☐ **no** ☐
These are non-essential foods and should be avoided during pregnancy.

10 Are you checking with a doctor or pharmacist before taking any medication?

yes ☐ **no** ☐

Take medication only when absolutely necessary, as some medications can be harmful to the developing baby (see page 176).

11 Are you drinking at least 1.5 litres (2½ pints) a day of water?

yes ☐ **no** ☐

Staying well hydrated is important for your metabolism during and after pregnancy, so get into the habit now of drinking plenty of fluids such as water and herbal teas.

12 Have you told your GP you are pregnant?

yes ☐ **no** ☐

It is better to do so sooner rather than later. In this way, any potential problems can be discussed and he or she can give you support and advice (see page 163).

your**score**

9–12 High scores are good news so many congratulations. Although nothing is guaranteed, you are doing everything you can to ensure that you stay healthy and support your baby's growth and development. Just try to keep up all your good habits and enjoy being pregnant – your baby will be here before you know it!

5–8 You have taken on board many of the things that will help give you a better chance of a healthy and successful pregnancy, but there is room for improvement. Use the questionnaire to identify areas of weakness and then read this step again to find out how to make changes to give yourself a better score.

0–4 You should reconsider the way in which you are approaching this first trimester, as it is the most important in terms of your baby's development and of your own health, not just now but after your pregnancy too. Re-read this step to find out how you can improve your score.

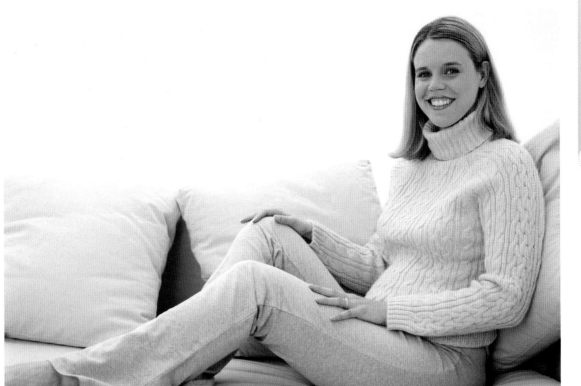

glossary

Amenorrhoea Absence of menstrual periods during a woman's reproductive years.

Amino acids Chemical compounds that are the building blocks of proteins.

Antioxidants Chemicals that neutralize the harmful effects of free radicals, which are molecules with the potential to damage body cells. Free radicals may be linked to cancers and heart disease.

Asthenozoospermia Inability of sperm to swim in a straight line or fast enough.

Azoospermia Absence of sperm in the seminal fluid due to obstruction, damage, or genetic abnormality.

Blastocyst A cluster of cells surrounding an inner cavity that develops at an early stage of pregnancy; the blastocyst embeds into the wall of the uterus and develops into an embryo.

BMI (body mass index) An indicator of the ratio of body fat to height. BMI is calculated by dividing a person's weight in kilograms by the square of his or her height in metres.

Carbohydrates Organic compounds, consisting of carbon, hydrogen, and oxygen, that are the body's main source of energy. Carbohydrates are obtained from a wide variety of foods, including grains and cereals, fruit, vegetables, and dairy products.

Chromosome A thread-like strand, found within the nuclei of all body cells, that carries genes – units of DNA that determine the physical characteristics and functions of the body.

Clomiphene A drug used to treat infertility in women who fail to ovulate.

Corpus luteum A small mass of tissue that develops from an empty egg follicle after the egg has been released at ovulation. It secretes the hormone progesterone, which helps prepare the uterus for pregnancy.

Donor eggs Eggs provided by one woman to be used by another in assisted conception procedures such as IVF.

Donor sperm Sperm donated by a man to be used in assisted conception procedures.

Dysmenorrhoea The medical term for painful periods.

Ectopic pregnancy Development of the embryo outside the uterus, nearly always in a fallopian tube.

Embryo The developing child in the uterus during its first eight weeks of life.

Endometriosis A disorder in which fragments of the lining of the uterus are found elsewhere in the body.

Epididymis One of two coiled tubes in the testes where sperm are stored prior to ejaculation.

Essential fatty acids Unsaturated fats, necessary for good health, that cannot be manufactured within the body and so must be obtained from food.

Fallopian tubes The two tubes that transport eggs from the ovaries to the uterus and where fertilization takes place.

Fertilization The union of an egg and a sperm, which results in the development of an embryo.

Fetus The developing child in the uterus from the end of the eighth week of pregnancy until birth.

Fibroids Non-cancerous tumours that develop in the wall of the uterus.

Follicle A sac within the ovary in which an egg develops.

FSH (follicle-stimulating hormone) A hormone produced by the pituitary gland in the brain that stimulates eggs to grow to maturity within their follicles in the ovaries.

Gamete The medical term for a sex cell (sperm or egg).

GIFT (gamete intrafallopian transfer) A technique for assisting conception in which a woman's eggs are removed from the ovary and mixed with sperm in the laboratory. The sperm and eggs are then placed in one of the fallopian tubes so that fertilization can take place naturally.

HFEA (Human Fertilisation and Embryo Authority) The body that licenses clinics to carry out assisted conception procedures such as IVF.

HSG *see* hysterosalpingogram.

Human chorionic gonadotrophin a hormone, produced by the placenta, that stimulates the ovaries to produce other hormones (oestrogen and progesterone), which are essential to a healthy pregnancy.

Hysterosalpingogram (HSG) an X-ray procedure in which liquid dye is squirted through the cervix to highlight the reproductive organs.

Hysteroscopy A technique for examining the uterus using a viewing instrument inserted through the vagina.

ICSI (intracytoplasmic sperm injection) An infertility treatment in which a single sperm is extracted from semen and injected into an egg to fertilize it.

IUI (intrauterine insemination) An assisted fertility treatment used to improve the likelihood of fertilization, in which sperm are introduced directly into the uterus using a catheter.

IVF (in vitro fertilization) A fertilization technique in which mature eggs are collected from an ovary and fertilized by sperm in the laboratory. Two or more of the eggs are then placed in the uterus.

IVM (in vitro maturation) A procedure in which immature eggs are collected from an ovary and allowed

to mature outside the body, before being fertilized by the same method used in IVF.

Laparoscopy Examination of the abdominal cavity using a viewing instrument inserted through a small incision in the abdominal wall.

LH (luteinizing hormone) A hormone produced by the pituitary gland that triggers the release of an egg at ovulation.

Menorrhagia The medical term for excessive menstrual bleeding.

Meridians Energy pathways, identified by acupuncturists, that pass through the major organs of the body.

Motility The ability of sperm to move and swim.

Morula The cluster of cells that develops from a fertilized egg during its journey down the fallopian tube to the uterus.

Oestrogen hormones The female sex hormones, which are responsible for the development and function of a woman's reproductive system and female characteristics, such as breasts.

OHSS *see* ovarian hyperstimulation syndrome.

OI *see* ovulation induction.

Oligomenorrhoea The medical term for an irregular menstrual cycle.

Oligozoospermia A low sperm count of below 20 million sperm per ml.

Ovarian hyperstimulation syndrome (OHSS) Overproduction of eggs following fertility treatment.

Ovulation The release of an egg (ovum) from the ovary, which occurs at midpoint in the menstrual cycle.

Ovulation induction (OI) Treatment with drugs (usually clomiphene) to stimulate production of the hormones that trigger ovulation.

Pelvic inflammatory disease (PID) Inflammation of the female reproductive organs, usually caused by infection.

Polycystic ovary syndrome (PCOS) A disorder in which multiple small cysts develop on the ovaries. PCOS can cause weight gain, unwanted hair growth, and infertility.

Progesterone A female sex hormone responsible for maintaining the function of a woman's reproductive system. Progesterone is produced by the corpus luteum, the tissue formed from the empty egg follicle after ovulation.

Sperm count The number of sperm per millilitre of semen.

Testosterone The male sex hormone, which is produced in the testes and is responsible for the development of male sexual characteristics.

Transfats Fats that are mostly produced by hydrogenation, a process used in the manufacture of vegetable fats commonly found in cakes, biscuits, pastry, and other prepared foods.

Trimester One of the three three-month developmental periods in pregnancy.

Trisomy A condition in which body cells have three copies of a particular chromosome instead of the normal two. Trisomies include developmental disorders such as Down's syndrome.

Ultrasound High-frequency sound waves used to produce images of body structures.

Varicoceles Varicose veins within the scrotum.

references

Page 13
■ Zadastra B M, Seidell J C, Van Noord P A H, te Velde E R, Habbema J D F, Vrieswijk B, Karbaat J (1993) Fat and female fecundity: prospective study of effect of body fat distribution on conception rates, *British Medical Journal* Vol 306, 484–7.

Page 16
■ Leridon H (2004) Can assisted reproduction technology compensate for the natural decline in fertility with age? A model assessment, *Human Reproduction* Vol 19, No. 7, 1548–1553.
■ Balen A, Jacobs H S (2003) *Infertility In Practice,* Churchill Livingstone p.18 and sources.

Page 17
■ Dunson D, Colombo B, Baird D D (2002) *Human Reproduction* Vol 17, No. 5, 1399–1403.

Page 18
■ Dooley M (2006) *Fit for Fertility,* Hodder & Stoughton p.242 and sources.

Page 24
■ Norman R J (2004) The potential danger of COX-2 inhibitors, *Fertility and Sterility* (American Society for Reproductive Medicine) Vol 81, No. 3, 493–4.

Page 42
■ Wilcox A J, Dunson D & Baird D D (2000) The timing of the "fertile window" in the menstrual cycle: day specific estimates from a prospective study, *British Medical Journal* Vol 321, 1259–1262.
■ Wilcox A J, Weinberg C R & Baird D D (1995) Timing of sexual intercourse in relation to ovulation, *New England Medical Journal* 333, 1517–1521.

Page 51
■ Wilcox A J, Weinbert C R & Baird D D (1995) Timing of sexual intercourse in relation to ovulation *New England Medical Journal* 333, 1517–1521.

■ **Page 52**
Balen A, Jacobs H (2003) *Infertility in Practice,* Churchill Livingstone p.284.

Page 55

■ Sheynkin Y et al (2004) Increase in scrotal temperature in laptop computer users, *Human Reproduction*.

■ Fejes I et al (2004) Study presented at European Society of Human Reproduction and Embryology Conference.

Page 78

■ Hassan M A M, Killick S R (February 2004) Negative lifestyle is associated with a significant reduction in fecundity, *Fertility and Sterility* (American Society for Reproductive Medicine) Vol 81, No. 2.

Page 80

■ (2007) Smoking and Reproductive Life, BMA.

Page 81

■ (2007) Smoking and Reproductive Life, BMA.

■ (2003) Patient Factsheet *Smoking and Infertility*, American Society for Reproductive Medicine.

■ Foster W (May 2005) *Human Reproduction*.

Page 80

■ Lloyd F H, Powell P, Murdoch A P (1996) Anabolic steroid abuse by body builders and male subfertility, *British Medical Journal* Vol 313, 100–101.

Page 89

■ Silveira E M, et al. (2007) Acute exercise stimulates macrophage function, *Cell Biochemistry Function,* Jan-Feb, 25(1), 63-73.

■ *Exercise and Immunity,* American College of Sports Medicine and sources.

Page 107

■ Dooley M (2006) *Fit for Fertility,* Hodder & Stoughton p.101 and sources.

■ ibid p.149 and sources.

Page 108

■ Hatch E E, Bracken M B (1993) Association of delayed conception with caffeine consumption, *American Journal of Epidemiology* 138 (12), 1082–1092.

Page 109

■ Lewith G (January 2007) Complementary Medicine Research Unit, University of Southampton, *The Times*.

■ Professor John Warner (January 2007) Imperial College, London, *The Times*.

Page 112

■ Thys-Jacobs S, Starkey P, Bernstein D, Tian J (1998) *The American Journal of Obstetrics and Gynecology* Vol 179, Issue 2, p444–452 and *The Journal of Women's Health*.

Page 122

■ (2005) *Zita West's Guide to Getting Pregnant,* Thorsons.

■ (2004) *Diaphragmatic Breathing,* The Cleveland Clinic Health System.

Page 134

■ Professor Sarah Berga (2006) Emory University, Georgia, USA, www.news.bbc.co.uk.

Page 137

■ Holt J (2001), Fertility Clinic, Derriford Hospital, Plymouth.

resources

resources

Zita West Clinic
37 Manchester Street
London W1U 7LJ
020 7224 0017
www.zitawest.com
Advice, treatments, and products to help couples take a
planned approach to fertility and pregnancy.

British Acupuncture Council (BAcC)
63 Jeddo Road
London W12 9HQ
020 8735 0400
www.acupuncture.org.uk

British Association for Counselling and Psychotherapy
BACP House, 15 St John's Business Park
Lutterworth
Leicestershire LE17 4HB
0870 443 5252
www.bacp.co.uk

The British Complementary Medicine Association (BCMA)
PO Box 5122
Bournemouth
Dorset BH8 0WG
0845 345 5977
www.bcma.co.uk

British Osteopathic Association
3 Park Terrace
Manor Road
Luton
Bedfordshire LU1 3HN
01582 488455
www.osteopathy.org

COTS (Childlessness Overcome Through Surrogacy)
Moss Bank
Manse Road
Sutherland

Lairg
IV27 4EL
01549 402777
www.surrogacy.org.uk

Endometriosis UK
50 Westminster Palace Gardens
Artillery Row
London SW1P 1RR
020 7222 2781
www.endo.org.uk

Fertility UK
Bury Knowle Health Centre
207 London Road
Headington
Oxford OX3 9JA
www.fertilityuk.org

Human Fertilisation and Embryology Authority (HFEA)
21 Bloomsbury Street
London WC1B 3HF
020 7291 8200
www.hfea.gov.uk

The Infertility Network UK
(INUK)
Charter House
43 St Leonard's Road
Bexhill-on-Sea
East Sussex TN40 1JA
08701 188088
www.infertilitynetworkuk.com

The International Institute of Reflexology
146 Upperthorpe,
Walkley
Sheffield
South Yorkshire
S6 3NF
01142 812100
www.reflexology-uk.co.uk

Manual Lymphatic Drainage UK
PO Box 14491
Glenrothes
Fife KY6 3YE
0844 800 1988
www.mlduk.org.uk

The Miscarriage Association
c/o Clayton Hospital
Northgate
Wakefield
West Yorkshire WF1 3JS
01924 200799
www.miscarriageassociation.org.uk

The Multiple Births Foundation
Hammersmith House Level 4
Queen Charlotte's & Chelsea Hospital
Du Cane Road
London W12 0HS
020 8383 3519
www.multiplebirths.org.uk

National Institute of Medical Herbalists (NIMH)
Elm House
54 Mary Arches Street
Exeter
Devon EX4 3BA
01392 426022
www.nimh.org.uk

QUIT (helping smokers to stop)
211 Old Street
London EC1V 9NR
020 7251 1551
Quitline 0800 00 22 00
www.quit.org.uk

The Society of Homeopaths
11 Brookfield
Duncan Close
Moulton Park
Northampton

Northamptonshire NN3 6WL
0845 450 6611
www.homeopathy-soh.org

Shiatsu Society
PO Box 4580
Rugby
Warwickshire CV21 9EL
0845 130 4560
www.shiatsusociety.org

Verity (The Polycystic Ovaries Syndrome self-help group)
Unit AS20.01
The Aberdeen Centre
22–24 Highbury Grove
London N5 2EA
www.verity-pcos.org.uk

useful websites

www.acebabes.co.uk (for families following assisted conception)
www.babycentre.co.uk
www.britishfertilitysociety.org.uk
www.nutrition.org.uk (British Nutrition Foundation)
www.daisynetwork.org.uk (Daisy Network Premature Menopause Support Group)
www.donor-conception-network.org
www.ein.org (European Fertility Network)
www.fertilityfriends.co.uk
www.fertilityuk.org
www.ivf.net
www.mothers35plus.co.uk
www.ngdt.co.uk (National Gamete Donation Trust)
www.relate.org.uk
www.repromed.co.uk (Centre for Reproductive Medicine)
www.rcog.org.uk (Royal College of Obstetricians & Gynaecologists)
www.tamba.org.uk (Twins & Multiple Births Association)
www.womens-health.co.uk

index

acknowledgments

Zita West would like to thank Jane Knight for her tremendous help, inspiration and support in the work at the clinic and in the writing of this book. Thanks also to Anita O'Neill, Brian Astley, Melanie Brown and Isobelle Obert. Special thanks to Deborah Beckerman for helping to put the words on paper and for her endless patience, Angela Baynham for her energy and support, and Esther Ripley and Sara Kimmins and all the creative team at DK.

DK would like to thank Deborah Beckerman for her generous editorial help, Ann Baggaley for proofreading and editing, Susan Bosanko for the index, Tara Woolnough and Zia Allaway for additional editorial assistance, and Niccy Kemp, Claire Legemah, Peggy Sadler and Simon Wilder for additional design assistance.

picture credits